Overcoming Abdominal Fat by Carmen Beese

Introduction

Belly fat is associated with a statistically higher risk of heart disease, hypertension, insulin resistance, and Diabetes Mellitus Type 2.

Relationship with diabetes
There are numerous theories as to the exact cause and mechanism in Type 2 Diabetes. Central obesity is known to predispose individuals for insulin resistance. Abdominal fat is especially active hormonally, secreting a group of hormones called adipokines that may possibly impair glucose tolerance.

Relationship with Alzheimer's Disease
A US study reported in May 2010 Annals of Neurology examining over 700 adults found evidence to suggest higher volumes of visceral fat, regardless of overall weight, were associated with smaller brain volumes and increased risk of dementia.

These are just the tip of the iceberg; abdominal fat can cause you many other health problems. Rid the abdominal fat is not only a matter of aesthetic; it is also a health matter.

Of course the aesthetic discomfort is the first to touch us. Throw the first stone, who never spent hours trying to find something to wear that would disguise the belly fat and ended up wearing something loose and unsexy? Or

2

just decided to dress in your favorite clothes just to have the 'waist growth' hanging out shouting to the world how unfit you are.

Everybody can lose abdominal fat! Achieving all you want in life is a matter of focus and knowledge. Everybody has the potential to become whatever they want in life. However, you need to know exactly what you have to do to get what you want. Lose abdominal fat is not that difficult and thousands of men and women achieved the bodies they wanted by following a plan that works.

Until you learn to eat right, take the right supplements, ignore the bad habits, know exactly how to exercise, you will have a very hard time trying to rid the abdominal fat.

Education is without doubt one of the best things you can do to help yourself get the best results. That is the reason why you should read this book very attentively. Here you will find the latest findings about body fat and how to achieve the body of your dreams.

Part 1: 30 Tips to Lose Stomach Fat

1. Food Types That Will Help You Lose Belly Fat

The right nutrients can help lose stomach fat for good and you can see the difference in the first week.

When thinking of getting rid of stomach fat it quickly comes to mind the terrible abdominal exercises. However, a good diet can also make a huge difference. Some celebrities use flaxseed. Rich in fiber, this cereal helps you to lose stomach fat and weight in general by increasing satiety and stimulating the bowels.

The accumulation of fat in the stomach area has several causes - physical inactivity, bad diet, genetic inheritance, psychological disorders and diseases such as hypothyroidism or constipation. The secret of a smaller waist is combining macronutrients (carbohydrate, protein, fat) with adequate intake of micronutrients (anything that is not macronutrient), in addition to regular exercise.

To lose stomach fat and get the tummy of your dreams, you will find here exactly what you have to eat and also when and how. It is vital to have small and varied meals throughout the day, avoiding the bad habit of snacking on caloric junk, especially simple carbohydrates. It is a complete nonsense to spend hours and hours without eating and during a single meal devour everything as if there will be no tomorrow. The ideal is to eat every four hours and adopt a balanced diet with aerobic exercise and healthy habits. This will enable you to lose up to 4cm in waist circumference over a month.

You must know how to choose the sources of fat, carbohydrate and protein. It is the quality of nutrients that help in the process of fat loss around the stomach area. Therefore, it is so important to eat the right food:

• **Rich in vitamin C:** blackcurrant, lemon, cherry, strawberry, orange, raw sweet pepper, mango, pineapple

• **Rich in beta carotene:** carrots, pumpkin, sweet potato, papaya, mango, star fruit, nectarine, peach, kale, chicory

• **Rich in vitamin B2:** greens color dark green (spinach, arugula, watercress, endive, escarole, chard), milk, lean meats (chicken), whole grains (oats, wheat, rye, rice, oatmeal, flaxseed , buckwheat)

• **Rich in vitamin D:** oily fish, liver, tuna, herring, Mackerel

• **Rich in catechins, bioflavonoids, polyphenols and antioxidants**: green and

5

white teas, which accelerate the metabolism, stimulate fat burning and acts as a diuretic

• **Rich in protein, minerals and vitamins A and D**: white cheese (cottage and ricotta), which are an important source of protein and work on the formation and repair of tissues

• **Rich in nutrients for rapid assimilation**: fruit juices with vegetables that require little effort digestive. For it to work properly eat them first thing in the morning.

• **Rich in fiber:** fruit and vegetables in general, which are sources of vitamins and minerals

• **White meat (chicken and fish)**: sources of protein with lower saturated fat, and some fish such as salmon, herring, sardines and mackerel are sources of omega 3 that helps increasing HDL (good cholesterol), preventing strokes.

Important Tips:

• Before lunch eat a salad plate. This helps give a feeling of satiety - you will eat less and lose stomach fat quicker

• Reduce fat, salt and sugar

• Replace industrialized ready made spices for natural herbs such as oregano, basil, parsley, coriander, onion, garlic, cinnamon, mustard, chilli, pepper and ginger extract. They don't contain sodium, which is very

6

good as it retains liquid.

• Replace soft and fizzy drinks to green and white teas. But avoid drinking during meals. This is very important tip to follow to lose stomach fat quicker.

• Red meat: Once a week maximum. Chicken and fish must be your choice for meat.

• Replace sausages, pepperoni, salami and chorizo for smoked turkey breast or Chester. But eat in moderation as they are a bit salty causing water retention.

• Food rich in fiber (whole grains, wheat and oat bran, flaxseed and rye flour, whole wheat bread, nuts and cake) minimize constipation. Just do not forget to increase water consumption. Otherwise the laxative effect of fiber becomes constipation causing the impression of excess abdominal fat.

• Avoid alcoholic drinks or just take it once a week because their high glycemic index won't help you to lose stomach fat.

• To combat the sedentary lifestyle, exercise more walking and cycling can be fun and a good start.

Lose stomach fat is not just aesthetical it is a health issue.

The benefits of making an effort to lose stomach fat, not only makes you feel good about yourself but also decreases the risk of diabetes, stroke and heart diseases.

2. Relax and sleep well

U.S. research has shown that stress causes hormonal changes that lead to increased rates of glucose in the blood stream. This causes the body to accumulate fat in the abdominal area.

3. Drink plenty of milk

Calcium can be a great ally in the fight against fat. A research at the University of Tennessee, USA, has shown that eating foods rich in calcium (milk, yogurt etc.) helps contain the hormone responsible for the accumulation of fat in the body.

4. Drink lots of white and green teas.

Eat all the berries. They have flavonoids that are known to fight the fat in the tummy area.

5. Put fiber on the plate

Everyone knows that the fibers keep the feeling of satiety for longer. This is because

8

they go through the digestive system a lot slower than other types of food. This decreases our desire to attack the fridge. You will find fiber in fruits, whole cereals, vegetables and also in beans.

6. Watch your posture

Always keep your shoulders open and spine straight. This decreases the impression of a prominent tummy. According to a U.S. study, a correct posture promotes an efficient blood circulation and helps to lose stomach fat. Avoid sitting more than 45 minutes straight. Take at least 2 minutes break and walk around.

7. Keep your hormones under control

Hormonal imbalances cause the accumulation of abdominal fat. At menopause, the situation worsens. The drop in oestrogen makes the distribution of fat irregular. This leads to the formation of stomach fat. After reaching 40 years old, do routine tests. This is the best way to find out hormonal problems.

8. Burn calories

Doing a physical activity is very important for anyone who wants to lose stomach fat.

9

Exercise speeds up metabolism and this increases the weight loss. It doesn't need to be something too demanding, just a 30 minute walk will do.

9. Willpower

This is the key ingredient for anyone who wants to lose stomach fat. To keep going with your diet and physical activities, you should focus on what it means to you to lose stomach fat. Think positive. When you feel like giving up, repeat to yourself: I have the discipline necessary to get where I want to be.

10. Gelatin An Important Ally To Lose Belly Fat

Nutritionists talk about the benefits of gelatin for health and beauty.

Tasty, refreshing and easy to prepare, gelatin has been treated for many years as a food for children. But after several studies, experts say that it brings health benefits to people of all ages, working, for example, as an important source of collagen, a protein that contributes to the strengthening of the nails, joints, hair and for moisturizing the skin.

Consumed regularly, gelatin aids in reducing levels of blood cholesterol, triglycerides and glucose control. This is good news if you are trying to lose belly fat because this simple food will have an important role in eliminating the bad fat in your body, especially around your stomach area. The food has properties that strengthen bones and prevents the body from diseases like osteoarthritis and osteoporosis. In addition, gelatin can help to retard the skin aging process.

According to research from several institutes, around the age of 25 our bodies begin to decrease the production of collagen and therefore, the substance must be found elsewhere. Combined with other foods, gelatin can greatly help in the fight against aging and stomach fat. With the high levels of collagen, the skin becomes firmer, manages to keep hydrated and is less likely to be marked by wrinkles while maintaining strong hair and nails.

There is a kind of gelatin that is far more effective than the normal ones. It goes by the name of hydrolyzed and is pumped with collagen. This protein is responsible for skin firmness and provides substances that accelerate the metabolism, in other words the burning of fat. By the age of 25 the body produces about 70% of collagen. Eventually, the body stops being able to keep itself from supporting the skin and the hair and nail strength. At the age of 50 the production falls to 30% of ideal. For this reason, the more powerful the gelatin, the better. The hydrolyzed is low in calories and, like the other, reduces hunger. It gives a feeling of fullness. This sends the information to the brain of satiety for longer. This product is incredibly powerful when trying to lose belly fat. See below the difference between these two types of gelatine.

Common Gelatin

It's a delicious and refreshing dessert. Therefore, it reduces anxiety and satisfies cravings for sweets.

Contains about 4.3% collagen, and the light version, 4.9%

Hydrolyzed Gelatin

Not a dessert. In addition to being consumed in powder form, there is a version in capsules.

Has an average of 85% collagen, 20 times more than conventional.

Remember that there are no miracles to make you lose belly fat. Do your part and use the tips as leverage. You have the choice and responsibility to lose belly fat not only for aesthetic reasons but mainly for health reasons.

11. Juice, Teas and Others

No miraculous formula has yet emerged to deliver the instant solution that we are so desperately looking for. However, it is proven that if we leave behind bad habits (for example, let laziness aside and walk 20 minutes a day) and focus on healthy solutions you will have your ultimate prize: a flat belly.

Here are some infallible solutions for you to lose stomach fat.

Fat Loss Juice

Ingredients
- 1 tablespoon of passion fruit
- 1 cup of cold centella asiatica tea
- 1 cup of water
- 30 ml liquid collagen protein supplement

Preparation
Blend everything in a blender and drink two or three times a day.

Teas

Olive Leaf Tea
The ideal is to drink three or four cups a day. If you have an 80cm waist you will lose an average of 8cm. Do not sweeten your tea. If you want to change the flavor, put in pineapple skin or a mint leaf.

Green tea
It speeds up your metabolism, burning fat. But do not exceed 800ml per day because you may experience heart burning and increased heart rate. Take after meals and in a warm temperature.

White bean flour

You can buy ready-made or do it in your own home (see recipe below). The white bean flour helps your body absorb less carbohydrate. It will also help to prevent diabetes and strengthen bones. Ideally take 1 tea spoon diluted in 100ml of water before all meals.

RECIPE

Preparation

- Wash 250g of raw white beans and let them dry in the sun
- Blend all in blender and then sift
- Put the flour in a jar for a week (note: for preserve the properties do not make more than 250g)

12. Ginger and Olive Oil

Ginger

This seasoning accelerates the metabolism and this increases the fat burning in the body. Eat a piece 2cm in length either raw, steamed or as tea three times a day.

Olive oil

Spanish and U.S. researchers have shown that olive oil has a special fat that combats the love handles that form in the stomach. Furthermore, this oil reduces bad cholesterol and prevents aging. Still, be careful of the calories and consume only 2 tablespoons every day.

13. Does Beer Prevent Me To Lose Stomach Fat?

You may have heard that beer makes you grow a nice and round belly, or even that beer is a diuretic. The expert answers our questions.

Yes! Unfortunately beer makes your belly grow bigger. Beverages stimulate the production of insulin, a hormone that promotes fat accumulation in the stomach. Due to the fact that beer has a low alcohol content, compared to wine and spirits, beer is often consumed in larger quantities, which means that you will ingest more calories and therefore accumulate fat around the stomach area.

If you are trying to lose stomach fat and are following a program, don't panic! You don't need to totally give up a beer with friends. You just need to decrease the amount. Another solution is to "dilute" the calories in the beer, alternating their use with other non-caloric beverages like water or soft light drinks.

After all, beer is good for the heart. According to scientific studies in different countries, the brew has a lot of B vitamins, and antioxidants - substances that help reduce bad cholesterol and raise good ones.

15

But to obtain these benefits, the dose should be moderate: a pint of beer, three times a week (four at most!). However, doctors warn those with gastritis, ulcers, diabetes, high triglyceride levels, history of alcoholism in the family or overweightness should not drink at all.

Save calories in the pub/bar and Lose Stomach Fat

Before you say no to happy hours, here are some tips for going out with friends that won't destroy your program to lose stomach fat.

· Take two cups of water for every glass of alcohol.

· Opt for lighter appetizers like lean cooked ham, olives, mix of seeds (sunflower seeds, nuts, peanuts – unsalted) and vegetable sticks.

How much you consume in calories each dose:
· Beer: 132 calories
· Wine white: 99 calories
· Wine Red: 109 calories
· Vodka and lemonade/coke: 220 calories
· Vodka: 120 calories
· Whiskey: 122 calories

Overcoming Abdominal Fat by Carmen Beese

14. Take These 5 Actions

After much research, the American nutritionist Susan Roberts realized that to control greed you just need to take five actions. Following her principles a group of volunteers managed to lose between 10 and 45 pounds without exercising.

Best of all: most of them did not put on weight again one year later. This successful method is in the book The Instinct Diet. For Susan, the big mistake is to try fighting the natural instinct to eat when you are hungry. Here you will find the following foolproof tricks to overcome greed, lose stomach fat and weight in general in a healthy way and ending the yo-yo effect. Start by following these tips today.

A. Choose foods that satiate more

Give preference to fiber and protein. These types of food satiate you which leads to pleasant feelings for longer. The best sources of protein are milk, fruits, cereals, yogurt, lean meats and green vegetables.

Supplement the diet with so-called good fats. They can be of vegetable origin – walnuts, peanuts, nuts, olive oil, canola oil or sunflower – or animal: especially tuna, salmon and sardines.

Choose wholemeal breads and pasta.

B. Do not take junk home

17

Keep yourself far way from candy, cookies, soft drinks and sausages. Keeping the kitchen cabinets full of junk food is the worst thing for those on a diet. In a moment of weakness, you will end up falling into temptation. These foods tend to be very attractive and loaded in flavor. This stimulates the brain and stomach to always ask for more. Therefore, escape them if you are serious about **lose stomach fat**!

C. Keep the food lean

Swap products for less calorie versions.

Replace deserts by fresh fruit salad and gelatin. Use the oven more than the frying pan. Thus, you avoid extra calories.

Replace full fat milk for skimmed, and chocolate for dried fruit.

Eat salad or vegetable soup before the main course (the vegetables cooked in the steam, keeping the nutrients).

Dilute orange juice with water.

The cheese fat is just enough so prepare sandwiches without margarine or mayonnaise.

D. Fight food boredom

To avoid getting bored of the food you are eating, vary the menu at every meal.

Overcoming Abdominal Fat by Carmen Beese

Diversification does not mean eating fattening foods! Search for new low calorie options, like a different fruit or cereal you have the habit of eating.

- Sprinkle quinoa or flaxseed on desserts or blend it in a smoothie.
- Prunes, lychees and apricots make a fabulous snack between meals.
- Always browse carefully in healthy shops, grocery stores and supermarkets to find other healthy foods with different tastes.

E. Reprogram your body now

Your brain just needs two weeks to get used to healthier foods. If you love fattening foods, it is because your brain is conditioned to wish for them every time you feel like eating.

For two weeks, train yourself to lose stomach fat and change your focus: whenever you feel hungry, eat something healthy. Soon, this choice will be easy and almost automatic.

Don't forget to drink two liters of water per day, plus teas, especially camomile, which is naturally calming and reduces hunger caused by anxiety.

15. Sesame Seeds Help You To Lose Stomach Fat

...And the Oscar goes to the double Calcium and Omega-3.

Sesame seeds are packed with these two nutrients which are well known for their properties to eliminate fat cells.

Including sesame paste or Tahini – as it is more commonly known – for breakfast every day gives a great help for anyone who wants to lose stomach fat and weight in general. You will see the scales pointer going down very quickly. Just a tablespoon of paste made with that seed on a slice of bread.

Study after study has shown that calcium not only interferes with the development of adipocytes – fat cells – but also stops the absorption of fat. So when the body lacks calcium we have an abundance in tummy and love handles. Not to mention that it also has a big role on the utilization of insulin, the hormone that regulates metabolism and hunger. If this substance – the insulin – is left free in the body, the increase in adipose tissue (fat) is clear and certain.

The role of omega-3 in the weight loss is less well known. It is known, however, that one of the functions of this fatty acid is to reduce inflammatory processes. What does this have to do with lose stomach fat? It's simple: when our body receives the unwanted visit of a micro-organism, the body builds up fat as a defence mechanism.

Of course, the body needs to store energy to get rid of the unwelcomed visitor. However, if the body is well supplied with omega-3, the risk of inflammation is quite small. Therefore, it is not necessary to store fat and the chances of you **lose stomach fat** is higher.

You can make your own paste or you can buy it ready.

Preparation:

Toast 1 cup of skinless sesame seeds. Let them cool and beat in a processor until it turns into paste.

16. Use the Magic Equation To Lose Stomach Fat

Without omitting bread and pasta from the menu, you can lose up to two pounds a week - the result appears mainly in the stomach area. The secret is to combine these food types with generous portions of lean protein and good fat.

The secret of the sure fire food combination to lose stomach fat:

The secret of this diet is to combine carbohydrates, protein and fat in all meals (from breakfast to dinner) to maintain hormone balance and keep burning fat constantly. Consumed in ideal proportions, protein and fat slow down the glycemic index of carbohydrates - it takes longer to be processed into sugar in the bloodstream and the production of insulin is kept in balance. When it is produced in excess, insulin causes the body to retain more fat and the effects can be sadly noted by the scales pointer.

The magic equation is as follows:
9 grams of carbohydrate = 1 C
7 grams of protein = 1 P
1.5 fat = 1 F

Together and in this proportion, the three nutrients **(1 C + 1 P + 1 F)** form a *block.*

So **(1 C + 1 P + 1 F) = 1 Block**

Depending on the meal, your plate should have one, two or three blocks. Complicated? Don't worry about counting the calories - in fact, forget it! The result - melt up to 2 pounds a week – it is entirely up to you. Best of all, the fat around your stomach area is the first to disappear.

The advantage of this diet is that you also learn how to select healthy carbohydrates, lean proteins and good fats.

This is another important rule: bad proteins and fat, such as butter and fatty meats, are left out. Instead opt for lean beef, chicken and fish which are food with less saturated fat (associated with cardiovascular disease and some types of cancer). The fish have an extra benefit: the omega, which helps prevent heart attacks and strokes. You will lose stomach fat while investing in your

Overcoming Abdominal Fat by Carmen Beese

health. Prefer wholemeal breads and pastas (carbohydrates rich in fibers) and the olive, almond and avocado (the good fat sources).

If you quench your thirst with soft drinks, stay away from them in the first two weeks: drink water but avoid sparkling at all costs, and moderate in fruit juice. During this period, avoid candy, desserts, chocolate and potato chips. They are on the list of foods with a very high glycemic index, which produce insulin spikes.

You can create your own diet:

Make your own menu with nine blocks per day, distributed as follows:

Breakfast: 2 C + 2 P + 2 F (2 blocks)
Morning snack: 1 C + 1 P + 1 F (1 block)
Lunch: 3 C + 3 P + 3 F (3 blocks)
Afternoon snack: 1 C 1 P + G + 1 (1 block)
Dining: 2 C + 2 P + 2 F (2 blocks)
and before bedtime: 2 F (here, the fat should be eaten alone and not counted as block).

In the tables below, pick your favorite foods:

Carbohydrates

Pineapple
Portion - 1 medium slice
Value - 1 C

Lettuce
Portion - 1 foot
Value - 1 C

White Rice
Serving size - 2 tablespoons
Value - 1 C

Brown rice
Serving size - 3 tablespoons
Value - 1 C

Asparagus
Portion - 12 stems
Value - 1 C

Plantain
Portion - 1 / 3 unit
Value - 1 C

Potato medium
Portion - 1 / 2 unit
Value - 1 C

Beetroot
Serving size - 2 tablespoons
Value - 1 C

Broccoli
Portion - 1 saucer plate
Value - 1 C

Carrot grated
Portion – 2 tablespoons
Value – 1 C

Canned peas
Serving size - 2 tablespoons
Value - 1 C

Overcoming Abdominal Fat by Carmen Beese

Beans
Portion – 3 tablespoons
Value - 1 C

Orange
Portion - 1 / 2 unit
Value - 1 C

Lemon
Serving Size - 2 units
Value - 1 C

Apples
Portion - 1 / 2 large unit
Value - 1 C

Pasta
Portion - 1 / 2 cup. (Tea)
Value - 1 C

Melon
Portion - 1 medium slice
Value - 1 C

Canned Corn
Portion - 1 tablespoon
Value - 1 C

Strawberry
Serving size - 4 units
Value - 1 C

Hearts of Palm
Serving size – 5 units
Value - 1 C

Brown Bread

Portion - 1 unit
Value - 1 C

French bread (inside included)
Portion - 1 unit
Value - 2 C

French bread crust only (without inside)
Portion - 1 unit
Value - 1 C

Pitta Bread small
Portion - 1 unit
Value - 1 C

Papaya
Portion - 1 / 4 unit (big)
Value - 1 C

Pear
Portion - 1 / 2 unit
Value - 1 C

Ravioli
Serving size - 6 squares
Value - 1 C

Arugula
Serving size - 2 packs
Value - 1 C

Orange juice
Portion - 1 / 3 cup
Value - 1 C

Apple juice
Portion - 1 / 3 cup

Value - 1 C

Grape Juice
Portion - 1 / 4 cup
Value - 1 C

Tomato
Portion - 1 unit
Value - 1 C

Grapes
Serving size - 6 units
Value - 1 C

Vegetables and fruit are carbohydrates.

Protein

Canned Tuna in water
Portion - 1 / 2 tin
Value - 1 P

Lean beef
Portion - 1 / 3 fillet (30g)
Value - 1 P

Egg
Serving Size - 2 units
Value - 1 P

Cottage cheese
Serving size - 2 tablespoons
Value - 1 P

Fish
Portion - 1 filet (75g)
Value - 1 P

27

Hamburgers
Portion - 1 unit (45g)
Value - 1 P

Chicken Breast
Serving size – 1 / 2
Value - 1 P

Turkey breast
Serving size - 2 slices (30g)
Value - 1 P

Ham lean
Serving size - 2 slices (30g)
Value - 1 P

Ricotta Cheese
Serving size - 3 tea spoons
Value - 1 P

Roast beef lean
Serving size - 2 slices (45g)
Value - 1 P

Salmon
Portion - 1 / 2 fillet (50g)
Value - 1 P

Sardines in water
Portion - 1 / 4 tin
Value - 1 P

Fats

Avocado
Portion - 1 tablespoon

Value - 1 F

Raw unsalted almonds
Serving size - 3 units
Value - 1 F

Raw unsalted peanuts
Portion - 5 units
Value - 1 F

Extra Virgin Olive Oil
Portion - 1 teaspoon
Value - 1 F

Black Olives
Portion - 1 unit
Value - 1 F

Green Olives
Serving size - 3 units
Value - 1 F

Food - Cream cheese light
Serving size - 2 teaspoons
Value - 1 F

Light Mayonnaise
Portion - 1 teaspoon
Value - 1 F

Soft Cheese Light
Portion - 1 teaspoon
Value - 1 F

Dairy*

Natural yoghurt

Portion - 1 (125 ml)
Value - 1 P + 1 C

Skimmed milk
Serving size - 1 cup (250 ml)
Value - 1 P + 1 C

Tofu
Portion - a thick slice
Value - 1 P + 1 C

* Check the labels: milk and dairy products
are high in carbohydrates.

Avocado – a word of warning
In excess it can make you put on weight and
also when consumed with sugar. In small
portions and eaten by itself, it could have the
opposite effect. It is a fruit rich in
polyunsaturated fat which, when taken at
bedtime intensifies the action of GH, the
growth hormone. In adults, it helps build
muscles and uses the stored fat for energy.

Tricks to lose stomach fat quicker:

• When eating a baked potato, add a filling
of chicken and light cream cheese. Despite
the increasing number of calories, chicken
(protein) and the cream cheese (fat) will
delay the processing of the potato
(carbohydrates) into sugar in the
bloodstream, maintaining balanced insulin
production.

- If you cannot resist the chocolate eat it within moderation and prefer those accompanied by almonds, which reduces the glycemic index of the chocolate.

- Another good combination: lean ham with melon and almond. The fruits are considered carbohydrate and therefore dramatically increase the amount of sugar in the blood. The turkey breast (protein) and almonds (fat) slow down this process.

- Alcoholic beverages have a high glycemic index. Replace sugar by sweeteners in cocktails and consume them together with protein food.

17. Lose Stomach Fat Knowing Your Metabolic Type

Find Out Your Metabolic Type And Lose Stomach Fat Quicker

For months you have eaten only half a slice of bread a day in an attempt to **lose stomach fat** and weight and nothing - the scale does not give the slightest hint that the effort is paying off. So pay attention: your metabolism can be the carbohydrate type. It means that your body needs more of this nutrient to work well and thus make you **lose stomach fat** more easily. Yes, you can eat bread and pasta without guilt.

Is your metabolic type protein? In this case,

31

meat and legumes should be a priority in your menu. There is also the mixed type, which asks for protein and carbohydrate in about the same proportion. Fat is also important in adequate quantity for this metabolic type.

Sorting metabolism types in three was the way specialists found to put together a diet close to the chemistry of our organism and increase our chances to **lose stomach fat** and weight.

Take the quiz and discover your metabolic type

Mark true or false based on what actually happens to you. Avoid thinking about what is right but you don't do. If in doubt skip or take some time to think.

Part 1

1. I am always hungry at breakfast time

2. At lunch, my appetite awakens

3. I got pretty hungry at dinner

4. I can not stay more than four hours without eating

5. Having a snack between meals makes me feel good

6. I think about food all the time

7. My energy levels improve when I eat meat or fish

8. A meal without meat does not satisfy my hunger

9. Meat or fatty foods give me energy

10. I can easily change sweet to salty

Add up all the false (F) answers and multiply them by 2. Do the same with the true (T) answers.

Part 2

1. I can not skip breakfast

2. Eating before bed improves my sleep

3. Drinking orange juice in the morning makes me sick

4. Only fruit does not satisfy me

5. Coffee makes me too energetic

6. My eyes and / or nose tend to become wet

7. I pass water quite a lot during the day

8. I have to cough frequently to clear my throat

9. I like to sleep until later in the morning

10. When I cut myself, the wound heals fast

Score 1 point for True and 1 point for false.

Results:

1. If the total of false answers is equal to or greater than 18, your metabolic type is **CARBOHYDRATE**.

2. If the total of true answers is equal to or greater than 18, your metabolic type is **PROTEIN.**

3. If the total of false answers is under 18 for both true and false, your metabolic type is **MIXED.**

Now that you know the test result, then you have to follow the menu corresponding to your type. It brings the ideal servings for carbohydrate, protein and fat, in addition it shows the items that can cause food allergy. Some food can cause cell inflammation, which contributes to weight gain. Avoid these foods during the diet, and ensure the success of your weight loss.

You may have answered some of the questions inappropriately and get a result that does not correspond to your metabolism type. So be aware of the signs below. If after 15 days you experience one or more of the items below, repeat the test and start the diet right for your type.

1. Continues to gain weight.

2. Has compulsion to certain foods.
3. Shows mood swings (depression, joy, euphoria ...).
4. If you feel weak, unwilling.
5. You are often with cold or flu.

Carbohydrate Type Metabolism

60% carbohydrate
25% protein
15% fat

You can eat generous portions of carbohydrate. But do not get them only from bread and pasta. This nutrient also should come from vegetables and fruit.

Option 1

Breakfast
• Fruit (1 medium slice of papaya or 1/2 persimmon)
• 2 slices of brown bread with unsweetened jam
• 1 pot of light yoghurt

Snack
• Fruit (1 pear or apple)
• 1 cup of chamomile tea

Lunch
• 1 plate of lettuce, arugula and tomatoes with 1 teaspoon of extra virgin olive oil
• 5 tablespoon of brown rice
• 2 tablespoon of beans
• 1 small fillet (80 g) of grilled fish

Snack
• 1 slice of brown bread with a thin slice
white cheese

Dinner
• 1 plate of steamed cabbage
• 4 tablespoons of brown of rice
• 1 small fillet (80g) of grilled chicken

Option 2

Breakfast
• Fruit (1 small banana or a slice of papaya)
• 1 cup of soy milk (coffee and sweetener,
optional)
• 2 full toast with light cream cheese

Snack
• Fruit (an apple or peach)

Lunch
• 1 plate of lettuce and watercress with 1
teaspoon of extra virgin olive oil
• 6 tablespoons of brown rice with carrots
and zucchini
• An omelette (2 egg whites with 1 slice of
turkey breast and onions)

Snack
• 1 light cereal bar

Dinner
• 1 plate of steamed broccoli
• 2 baked potatoes with herbs, leeks and 2
teaspoons of extra virgin olive oil
• 1 small fillet (80 g) of fish

Option 3

Breakfast
• 1 / 2 papaya with 2 tablespoons of oatmeal
• 1 cup of skimmed milk (coffee and sweetener, optional)

Snack
• Fruit (a pear or two figs)
• 2 salt and water crackers with 2 slices of white cheese

Lunch
• 1 plate of lettuce and cucumber with a teaspoon of extra virgin olive oil
• 6 tablespoons of wholemeal pasta with tomato sauce
• 2 tablespoons of squash steamed
• 1 small fillet (80 g) of fish roasted with mushroom

Snack
• 2 wholemeal toast with cottage cheese

Dinner
• 2 tablespoons of steamed zucchini with 1 teaspoon of extra virgin olive oil
• 4 tablespoons of rice
• 1 small fillet (80g) grilled chicken

What to avoid

Red meat, milk, beans and lentils in excess. These foods are a source of purines, a type of protein that can cause food allergy in carbohydrate types.

Overcoming Abdominal Fat by Carmen Beese

Protein Type Metabolism

30% carbohydrate
40% protein
30% fat

Extra doses of protein and fat are essential for this type, but it is important that these nutrients come from lean meat, grains and nuts.

Option 1

Breakfast
• 2 slices wholemeal bread with 2 tablespoons hummus
• 1 cup (250 ml) of skimmed milk (coffee and sweetener, optional)

Snack
• Fruit (1 small apple)
• 1 handful of nuts (almonds or walnuts)

Lunch
• A saucer plate of arugula and cherry tomatoes with 1 tablespoon of extra virgin olive oil
• A small cup of wholemeal pasta with mozzarella
• 2 tablespoons of cooked soybeans
• 2 chicken thighs (120 g) skinless roasted

Snack
• 1 pot of light yoghurt (sweetener, optional)

Dinner

- a saucer plate of steamed cauliflower with a tablespoon of extra virgin olive oil
- 3 tablespoons of brown rice with almonds
- 1 large slice (120 g) lean pork roast

Option 2

Breakfast
- 2 wholemeal toasts with a scrambled egg
- 1 cup (250 ml) soy milk beaten with 3 tablespoons of avocado (optional sweetener)

Snack
- 4 almonds (or 2 Brazil nuts)

Lunch
- a saucer plate of cabbage and tomato with extra virgin olive oil
- 4 tablespoons of cooked quinoa (or mince soya)
- 1 large fillet (120 g) of fish

Snack
- a protein bar

Dinner
- a saucer plate of cooked green beans with 1 teaspoon of extra virgin olive oil
- 1 tablespoon of brown rice
- 2 tablespoons of beans
- 4 pieces (120 g) of lean beef

Option 3

Coffee Morning
- 2 slices wholemeal bread with 2 slices of white cheese and 2 slices of turkey breast

- 1 pot of light yoghurt

Snack
- Fruit (an apple or pear)
- 4 almonds (or 2 Brazil nuts)

Lunch
- a saucer plate of watercress and grated carrot with 1 tablespoon of extra virgin olive oil
- 3 tablespoons of brown rice
- 3 tablespoons of beans
- 1 big steak (120 g) fillet mignon in Madeira sauce

Snack
- 1 cup (200 ml) of skimmed milk beaten with 1 tablespoons of protein powder (whey protein type) and two prunes

Dinner
- a saucer plate of steamed eggplant with a tablespoon of extra virgin olive oil
- 2 tablespoons of brown rice
- An omelette (2 eggs and 2 slices medium white cheese)

What to avoid
Especially sweets and refined flour products. There are foods that accelerate the production of the insulin hormone, famous for favoring the storage of fat in all kinds metabolism. But the damage in protein types is even greater.

Metabolism Mixed Type

50% carbohydrate
30% protein
20% fat

You can eat carbohydrates, protein and fat in more balanced proportions. Choose healthier sources: pastas and whole grains, lean meats and good fats.

Option 1

Breakfast
• Fruit (1 medium slice of avocado or papaya
• 1 cup. (Tea) of skimmed milk (coffee and sweetener, optional)
• 2 full toast with cottage cheese

Snack
• Fruit (1 slice of pineapple, melon or watermelon)

Lunch
• 1 plate lettuce with grated beets and carrots with 1 tablespoons of extra virgin olive oil
• 1 and 1 / 2 big pasta spoons of wholemeal pasta with ricotta
• 1 medium drumstick (80g) roasted (no skin)

Snack
• a light fruit yogurt

Dinner
• 3 tablespoons of fresh peas steamed
• 3 tablespoons of brown rice
• 2 tablespoons of chick-peas cooked

- 1 medium fillet (100 g) of fish grilled with mustard sauce

Option 2

Breakfast
- 1 cup green tea or fennel
- 2 wholemeal bread toast with 2 slices of turkey breast

Snack
- 1 pot of light yoghurt milk

Lunch
- 1 plate of lettuce, tomato and olives with 1 teaspoon of extra virgin olive oil
- 1 plate of steamed broccoli
- 4 tablespoons of brown rice
- 2 tablespoons of lentils
- 1 medium chicken breast (100g) grilled

Snack
- 1 slice of wholemeal bread with light cream cheese

Dinner
- 1 plate of lettuce and arugula with 1 teaspoon of extra virgin olive oil
- 1 medium wholemeal pita bread
- a small portion (80 g) strips of grilled beef

Option 3

Breakfast
- 1 cup (250 ml) of soya milk blended with two prunes
- 2 slices of wholemeal bread with light

cream cheese

Snack
• Fruit (1 small banana or peach)
• 2 Brazil nuts

Lunch
• 1 plate of watercress and arugula with 1 teaspoon of extra virgin olive oil
• 4 tablespoons of rice
• 3 tablespoons of beans
• 1 / 2 eggplant stuffed with mince beef

Snack
• 4 dried apricots
• 1 pot of light yoghurt

Dinner
• 1 plate of palmito and tomatoes with 1 teaspoon extra virgin olive oil
• 3 tablespoons of carrot puree
• 1 small fillet (80 g) of fish grilled with mushrooms

What to avoid
Breads and pastas rich in gluten. This protein is difficult to digest, therefore, is related to indigestion and food allergy in the mixed type.

18. Lose Stomach Fat Eating Food Rich in Water

Everybody knows it's important to drink plenty of water. But instead of just putting the liquid in the glass, fill your plate with it!

Overcoming Abdominal Fat by Carmen Beese

A survey done in the United Sates showed that food rich in water are most effective for those who want to lose stomach fat and weight. This is because these foods have the power to remove the fat, especially around the stomach area.

The researchers studied two groups of overweight individuals who consumed the same number of calories. One group ate more food with high water content. After six months, people in that group eliminated about 2 pounds more than the group who had a more dry diet.

But the biggest benefit was: the high content water diet group lost on average twice more around the stomach area. A diet rich in water content definitely helped the group of individuals to lose stomach fat quicker. This happened because the water food helps lower blood sugar levels and reduces the amount of insulin. When insulin goes down, the body begins to burn its fat stores. And it starts just in the right place – the stomach area.

According to specialists in nutrition food with lots of water help to **lose stomach fat** and weight in general because they quench the stomach, reducing appetite. Fruit and vegetables are rich in water and facilitate the work of the kidneys, which eliminate the liquid retained more efficiently. Fruit, incidentally is the champion: about 80% of its composition is water.

Overcoming Abdominal Fat by Carmen Beese

Rich water content food that will help you to **lose stomach fat:**

Fruit: pear, apple, melon, watermelon, avocado, banana, mango
Vegetables: cucumber, celery, watercress, carrot, beet

19. Smoothies that take the hunger away and help you lose stomach fat and weight

Meet three home made smoothies that end up with cravings for sweets, accelerate the metabolism and help you to lose 5 lbs of body fat per week.

It is the chocolate milkshake created by nutritionists. It takes away the hunger, the craving for sweets, speeds metabolism and burns fat. Coupled with a 1,200 calories menu it will eliminate up to 2 kg per week with the additional benefit of flaxseed, your hair and skin will improve significantly.

Chocolate milkshake

Ingredients
- 1 cup (200 ml) yogurt
- 2 spoons (soup) of oatmeal (prolongs the feeling of fullness and accelerates the burning of fat)

- 1 spoon (soup) of ground golden flaxseed (is good for the heart and gut, and leave skin and beautiful hair)
- Sucralose sweetener (to taste)
- 1 spoon (tea) cocoa powder (it has antioxidant effect and combat premature aging)
- 1 large banana (energy, being high in fiber and potassium)

Way of doing
Beat all ingredients in blender. If desired, add ice.

Berry Smoothie

Ingredients
- 1 spoon (soup) shredded coconut
- 100 ml light soy milk
- 100 g yogurt
- 1 spoon (soup) filled with quinoa flakes (speeds up metabolism and controls the production of insulin)
- 1 cup (tea) of red fruits, like blackberry, blueberry and strawberry (has anti-aging effect and enhances satiety)

Way of doing
Beat all ingredients in blender. If desired, add ice.

Fruit Smoothie

Ingredients
- 1 slice of pineapple (speeds up metabolism and burn calories by up to 30%)
- 1 / 2 mango
- 1 / 2 small avocado
- 100 ml white tea
- 1 spoon (soup) of oatmeal (prolongs the feeling of fullness and accelerates the burning of fat)
- 1 cup (200 ml) fat free yogurt (accelerates the weight loss process and hinders the formation of fat)

Way of doing
Beat all ingredients in blender. If desired, add ice.

20. Pumpkin A powerful Weapon to Lose Stomach Fat

With 90% of its pulp made of water, the pumpkin has few calories but enough vitamins to help you eat well without piling fat around your stomach.

Eating something tasty that goes well in most dishes and is not fattening is just like a dream for the ones who are trying to lose stomach fat.

It is so low in calories that 100 grams of cooked pumpkin has only 20 calories. Moreover, it is extremely healthy. Rich in minerals and vitamins it has beta-carotene, which reduces the risk of cancer and heart

47

disease. For all that, it is an indispensable ingredient in a balanced diet.

You can make use of every bit of the pumpkin. See how each piece of plant can be used in cooking:

- The Flesh
It gives an amazing flavor to sweet and savory dishes, like soups, jams and stews. The combination with beef is mouthwatering. You can also use it on gnocchi (see recipe below) and pancakes.

- Skin
Cooked with rice and mince beef it gives a special flavor.

- Seeds
Just toast them for about 12 minutes and you will transform them into a healthy snack.

Health benefits

- Prevents disease
The pumpkin is rich in beta carotene, a substance that prevents cancer, strokes, cataracts and heart disease.

- Balances Cholesterol
Fiber and water help to eliminate fat and regulate the gut which is fantastic when trying to lose stomach fat.

- Essential minerals
Pumpkin seeds are a source of iron, zinc, phosphorus, potassium and magnesium.

These minerals have an important role in fat loss.

- Revitalize the skin
It has vitamin B3, which stimulates collagen formation leaving your skin smooth and healthy. It also avoids problems with digestion.

Pumpkin Gnocchi

2 pounds of pumpkin
2 eggs
4 cups (tea) of flour
4 tablespoons margarine
4 tablespoons of grated cheese (optional)

HOW TO PREPARE:

Cut the pumpkin into pieces, remove the skin and seeds. Cook it well. Drain the water, mash with a fork. Add the eggs, milk, flour and salt to taste, mix well until making a consistent dough. Make flat cakes and cook in boiling water, removing them as soon as they float on the water. Arrange the gnocchi on a plate and season with melted butter and grated cheese (optional). Alternatively, cover with tomato sauce.

Pumpkin Pancake

Ingredients

1 cup (tea) milk
3 eggs

½ cup (tea) pumpkin cooked and squeezed
4 tablespoons of flour
1 tablespoon of oil
A pinch of salt
Oil for greasing the pan

Filling:
4 teaspoons olive oil
1 medium onion, chopped
2 cloves garlic, minced
 ½ kg mince chicken
1 tomato, peeled and seeded, chopped
½ cup (tea) cream cheese
½ cup chopped parsley
Salt to taste

How to prepare

Beat the ingredients in a blender until the
dough is smooth
Place a portion of this mixture into a greased
pan and spread to form a round pancake
Let it cook on both sides
Repeat with the remaining dough
Reserve.
Heat the oil in a pan and fry the onion and
garlic
Add the chicken and fry it
Then add the tomatoes, parsley and salt, stir
for another 5 minutes on medium heat
Add the cream cheese
Mix well
Fill the pancakes
Serve them with the sauce of your choice.

21. Fruits that help to lose stomach fat

Pear is on that team and oranges as well. How so? Isn't it full of calories? Yes, but...

Pear

It has its merits and not just the popular apple - in time to wipe away those extra pounds. Research Institute of Social Medicine, University of Rio de Janeiro - and published in the Journal of Nutrition, one of the most respected American magazines about nutrition - showed that women who ate three pears a day for 12 weeks consumed fewer calories and lost more weight than those that had no fruit at all. The study was conducted with 411 volunteers aged between 30 and 50 years. The pear has the great advantage of being very fibrous. Concentra, on average, 3 grams of dietary fiber per 100 grams - almost double the apple, which provides 1.6 grams. Furthermore, consumption of one unit represents 12% of the daily requirement of fiber, which is about 25 grams per day. They are also a great source of insoluble fiber, which are related to the prevention of constipation and diseases like diverticulitis and colon cancer, complete Tania.

Grapefruit and 'sisters'

Want a reason to revere this fruit? Eating half a grapefruit or its juice taken before each meal may help in losing up to a pound a week, even if you do not change anything in your diet. That was the conclusion reached by researchers at the Scripps Clinic in California, a network of non-profit health and investing heavily in education. They followed 100 obese people for 12 weeks. After this period, it was found that components of the fruit help regulate the production of insulin, a hormone that is intimately connected to the storage of fat. Low levels of insulin also contribute to ward off hunger for longer when the rates are high, the hormone stimulates the hypothalamus, the brain region that, among other functions, regulates hunger. They contain the same compounds and act the same way in weight loss, guaranteed.

Green Banana

Truth. At this stage, it makes the scale to render thanks to a resistant starch that is present even in full pasta in white beans, the lentil, barley and whole grain bread, which are very powerful sources of satiety. This effect was more than proven in a U.S. survey by Louisiana State University and published in the Journal of Obesity. According to the study, this starch stimulates hormones that make the body feel satisfied and signal it's time to stop eating. Resistant starch also causes an increase in intestinal peristalsis, which may decrease the absorption of nutrients and, therefore, calories. Another fact: a small study from the University of Colorado revealed that the burning of fat was 23% higher among patients that included foods rich in starch. Can you eat green bananas? Yes, you will find great recipes on the Internet.

22. Eggplant Water

Discover the incredible benefits of eggplant water! It helps reduce stomach fat, cellulite, lose weight and even fights cholesterol.

Eggplant is a versatile food. No wonder it became one of the main ingredients in world cuisine. Eggplant is tasty, has a fundamental role in maintaining health and has a major influence on weight loss!

Eggplant helps you to lose stomach fat, regulates the intestine functions and lowers cholesterol.

Why is the eggplant good?

A good diet requires the ingestion of 25-30 grams of fiber daily. The eggplant is great in that sense, because it has very high concentration of fiber: a unit of 150g contains about 4.35g of fiber - not to mention the other benefits.

Check all the advantages of both types of fiber contained in eggplants:

Insoluble fiber

Present mainly in raw eggplant, this kind of fiber takes longer to be eliminated from the stomach, which delays the feeling of hunger. Result: you end up eating less and thus eat fewer calories.

Soluble fiber

They are the great secret eggplant water, as they come off the food as it gets soaked. The water then becomes rich in these soluble fibers, which in the body turns into a kind of gel capable of absorbing fat and eliminating it. You will lose stomach fat more easily.

The benefits of eggplant

A. Helps lose stomach fat

Eggplant has a substance called saponin, which acts as a detergent: breaks the molecules of fat in the blood and prevents the body from absorbing it. This means you can lose the fat around your waist quicker.

B. Fight cellulite

Eggplant has anti-inflammatory substances that work miracles to reduce cellulite, since the "holes" are nothing more than an inflammation of the cells, aggravated by eating fat foods.

C. Prevents diseases

Being full of phenolic compounds - antioxidants - the eggplant reduces free radicals that attack cells. Thus, it protects the organism from diseases like cancer. It also reduces the aging process.

D. Improves Bowl Functions

The fibers in the fruit act as a natural laxative, regulating the intestines and improving digestion. Thus the whole body becomes healthier and reduces your stomach size significantly. Yes it is a fruit not a vegetable as many people think!

Eggplant Water

Cut eggplant in half cubes. Leave the pieces to soak in 250 ml of water overnight. Insoluble fiber will be released in the water making this water incredibly powerful. Early the next morning, take a drink on an empty stomach without sieving.

To vary the recipe, beat half eggplant with half orange juice and drink during the day.

Other fruit that will help you to lose stomach fat:

There are more foods full of fiber, which are great for removing fat, according to nutritionists:

Pineapple: 1 medium slice - 1.10 g fiber
Dried black plum: 4 units - 0.51 g fiber
Banana: 1 medium - 2.40 g fiber
Guava: 1 medium - 5.04 g fiber
Orange: 1 medium - 2.60 g fiber
Apple with skin: 1 unit - 3.50 g fiber

23. Calcium: Important Weapon To Lose Stomach Fat

Increasingly, obesity has been recognized as a problem of multifactorial origin, which is involved in environmental, nutritional, physiological and genetic factors. Within this complexity, current scientific studies point to factors more specific in trying to find solutions to this public health problem.

It was during one such study, an effect that "anti-obesity" of calcium from dairy products was observed. This research has shown that higher intake of calcium (between 400-1000mg/day) through the ingestion of two cups of yogurt daily, produced a decrease in blood pressure accompanied by a decrease of 4.9 kg in body fat.

The explanation would be in the action of the hormones (1,25 (OH) 2D and 1,25 (OH) 2D3), responding to lower calcium intake and exercise effects on lipid metabolism, increasing lipogenesis and decreasing lipolysis.

The action of the hormone 1,25 (OH) 2D3 receptor occurs in the adipocyte, where there is inhibition of UCP2 protein, responsible for lipid oxidation. Without oxidation, lipogenesis occurs and the formation of adipocytes and fat.

The agouti gene is the factor responsible for lipogenesis and increased adiposity. However, when there is increased intake of calcium, hormones of calcium metabolism (1,25 (OH) 2D, 1,25 (OH) 2D3) are suppressed to control the negative feedback. The lipogenesis is inhibited and lipolysis occurs. Then, the lipid accumulation is avoided, and the percentage of fat decreases.

These studies were conducted primarily on mice and then in different populations (young women, elderly, children, lactose intolerant, and obese). The results are itemized below:

- A study with two groups of rats, where a group ate little calcium and others ate the recommended amounts and increasing calcium and dairy products. Mice that did not ingest amounts of calcium suffered mass gain and body fat, whereas the group of rats that ingested calcium or dairy products showed loss of body mass 26-40%, and there was caloric restriction in their diet. It was also noted that lipolysis was further stimulated in rats that ate dairy products as a source of calcium, compared with animals who obtained calcium through supplements.

- Another study indicated an inverse relationship between calcium intake and glucose tolerance. This study demonstrated that there is no loss of weight or body fat between glucose intolerant, and the reason is still being studied.

57

- A third report said the largest amount of calcium intake and physical exercise causes a further increase in lipid oxidation. They are a 10% higher compared with the diet rich in calcium but without physical activity.

- Among the obese or overweight individuals, it was noted that those who consumed more dairy products had lower incidence and risk of developing insulin resistance. In addition, individuals who participated in the study lost body mass and decreased their percentage of body fat.

- A more recent and larger, evaluated the benefits of calcium and dairy on body mass control. Study participants were 32 obese subjects, who started the study following a reduced calorie diet. Gradually, were added to the diet supplements of calcium, with the amount varying between 400-500mg/dia. Days later, calcium supplementation was increased to 800mg daily intake of 3-4 servings of dairy each day (equivalent to 1,200 mg / day). All obese subjects showed loss of body weight every time they increased the calcium supplementation. However, at the end of six months, the group of people who ate dairy products lost more body mass than those who were supplemented with calcium. It was noted, again, the largest dairy in the loss of efficiency and control of body mass in hypocaloric diets (6).

What region of the body is there greater fat loss with diets high in calcium?

After undertaking a study conducted by Zemel (6), we observed a greater loss of fat in the trunk, formed by the abdomen and chest. The loss of body fat in this region with a reduced calorie diet was 19%, and the result after the same diet supplemented with calcium was 50%. There was also a greater loss when calcium was obtained through the ingestion of dairy products (66%) (6).

Why dairy products are more effective than calcium supplementation, when the goal is the loss of body mass?

It is believed that other components of dairy products are also involved in the benefit attributed to calcium. However, further studies are needed for this statement to be concrete.

We know, therefore, that the presence of calcium in the diet, mainly through the ingestion of dairy products (3-4 servings), produces an effect "anti-obesity" through various reactions, inhibiting or stimulating the lipid metabolism. The various observational studies in animals and humans show us that fat loss and weight are real and visible every time the intake of calcium increases.

Once again we are shown the importance of calcium in our diet through the ingestion of

59

dairy products, which are important sources of this mineral.

24. Eggplant flour The Secret To Lose Belly Fat

Learn about all the properties of eggplant flour and see how to lose stomach fat and weight, adding this product to your diet.

Eggplant flour shrinks the tummy and helps you to lose weight! This good news is the result of a study.

How did they get this information? For 60 days, a group of volunteers aged between 30 and 45 years added to a low-calorie diet, 4 tablespoons of eggplant flour. Also during this period, other women did the same scheme, but without consuming the product.

Conclusion: who ate the flour lost 13 lbs and 4.7 in waist. The ones who did not, lost 6 lbs and 1.2 inches around the waist.

The benefits of eggplant flour

A. Makes you lose stomach fat

The flour combined with a diet low in calories will burn body fat, especially in the abdominal area. With the decrease in visceral fat, you will eliminate the risk of diabetes type 2.

B. Weight Loss
According to nutritionists the niacin, vitamin

60

present in eggplant - acts in the biochemical reactions responsible for the metabolic processes that make you lose weight.

C. Reduces levels of LDL cholesterol
With the acceleration of intestinal transit, bile salts (Substances that help in digestion of fat) are not absorbed by the body. To rebuild them, the body uses LDL (bad fat) and thus reduces its concentration.

D. Improves intestinal transit
As the fibers are not absorbed by the body, they promote increased stool and regulates the bowel. However, the consumption of flour should be associated with increased water intake to balance the bowel.

E. Take your hunger away
The soluble fiber found in eggplant flour, absorbs water from the body and when in the stomach it increases in size.

Conclusion: The body tells the brain that the body is satiated and no longer needs to be fed in the coming hours.

F. It has diuretic action
Rich in B vitamins, eggplant flour promotes the proper functioning of the kidneys.

G. Assists in the treatment of arthritis and rheumatism
The product helps reduce the concentration of uric acid in the body, excess blood accumulates in the form of crystal and

Overcoming Abdominal Fat by Carmen Beese

causes joint pain.

Make your eggplant flour at home:

Preparation
In a baking dish, place 1 kg of eggplant unpeeled and cut into slices. Then bake at a temperature of 200 º C for about 2:15 hrs or until crisp and dried.

Now put the eggplant in the processor blender to powder.

- Amount: 100 g.
- Storage: Store the flour in a jar and seal it. Keep it in a fresh place and away from light. It may be kept in the refrigerator.
- Validity: about a year.

25. Three natural remedies that help lose stomach fat and weight naturally and inexpensively

A flat tummy is the dream of almost every woman. But liposuction does not fit into any pocket (not counting any risks and health issues a surgery involves.) Thanks to the evolution of herbal medicines today with a little willpower you can say goodbye to stomach fat and love handles safely and inexpensively.

Because they are natural, almost anyone can use the pills, except for children, pregnant women who are breastfeeding and the elderly. Here are the substances that cause an effect of liposuction on your figure.

End the lion hunger:

- Use: Caralluma Fimbriata, a species of cactus found in the region of Africa, India, Arabia, southern Europe and Afghanistan.

- Advantages: It is considered one of the best appetite suppressants because it increases the feeling of satiety. Furthermore, no side effects - ie, nothing to spend a sleepless night, waking up grumpy or sink into depression.

Accelerate your metabolism:

- Use: Citrus aurantium, bitter orange extract.
- Advantages: Turns your metabolism, promoting greater energy expenditure. It also burns fat, prevents indigestion and increases the provision as it stimulates the release of adrenaline. Also protects you from insomnia and risks of heart attack and stroke.

Cut the pounds of bread, pizza and macaroni:

- Use: Phaseolamin (phaseola vulgaris), extracted from the beans.

- Advantages: Reduces the absorption of carbohydrates, fat burning localized and improves the functioning of the intestine.

26. Eat 5-6 meals per day

Consumption of food involves the digestion of food and absorption of nutrients (proteins, carbohydrates and fats). Digestion and absorption require energy to occur. Thus, food intake causes the body to expend energy to support the digestion and absorption.

The increased frequency of food intake throughout the day will increase your body's metabolism for the following two main reasons:

Your body will be forced to increase the daily energy expenditure due to frequent activation of the processes of digestion and absorption induced by food intake many times throughout the day. Eating is often perceived by the body as a sign of energy / food abundance.

Because of this, the body will increase energy expenditure (increased metabolic rate), since there is no need for frequent intake those calories are stored as energy stores (as fat in adipose tissue of fat), what happens during the hunger state (which occur during periods of food deprivation).

From one point of view of hormone, the

Overcoming Abdominal Fat by Carmen Beese

abundance of food (represented by an increased frequency of food intake) causes an increase in thyroid hormone (T3 and T4) secretion - that ultimately determines how much it will increase metabolism.

Remember high levels increase the metabolism of thyroid hormones, low levels of thyroid hormones depress the metabolism leading to fat gain!

If you pay attention, fat people are usually those who split their daily diet to no more than 2-3 meals! This frequency of meals puts the body into a starvation / deprivation of food, so the body responds by decreasing the metabolism through the reduction of thyroid hormones!

The highest frequency of daily food consumption is one of the easiest and most natural weapon we have in our hands to manipulate and improve the secretion of thyroid hormones and thus to increase the body's metabolism!

Thus, fat loss arising from the increased frequency of daily food intake is best represented schematically by the following events:

A. Increased frequency of food intake.
B. Plenty of food.
C. Increased secretion of thyroid hormones.
D. Increased metabolic rate.
E. Increased fat loss.

Overcoming Abdominal Fat by Carmen Beese

27. Consume foods rich in protein at each meal to increase metabolism

For each of your daily meals, be sure to include foods that contain high quality proteins (chicken, eggs, protein powder, red meat, fish), if your goal is to increase your metabolism!

Proteins are three times higher among all other nutrients (carbohydrates and fats). DIT represents the dietary induced thermogenesis.

Explanation: all the nutrients (proteins, carbohydrates and fat), requires energy to be digested by the gastrointestinal tract and then absorbed into the bloodstream. The energy the body burns to digest and absorb nutrients is called DIT.

DIT is different for each nutrient:

DIT for protein is 25%
DIT for carbohydrate is 5%
DIT for fat is 2%

Let's do a practical example to understand this concept better.

Expenditure of body energy to digest proteins:

Overcoming Abdominal Fat by Carmen Beese

100g tuna in water contains approximately 25g of protein.
Each gram of protein has a caloric value of 4 kcal.
The total consumption of calories per 100g of tuna is therefore about 100 kcal (25g protein x 4 kcal = 100 kcal).

So in terms of numbers of the body's energy expenditure to digest and absorb protein from 25g to 100g tuna is 25kcal:

As you can see the consumption of protein increases the body's energy expenditure more than other nutrients. This explains why it is important to introduce them in each of the daily meals, if the objective is to increase the body's metabolism, which ultimately represents the key factor to lose stomach fat and weight guaranteed.

28. Eating carbohydrates with a low glycemic index

The glycemic index (GI) is the rate at which a carbohydrate contained in food is converted into glucose (simple sugar) and enters the bloodstream.

Thus, the higher the GI of a carbohydrate the faster it enters the bloodstream, the lower its GI slower than it enters the bloodstream.

Carbohydrates trigger insulin secretion. The

faster a carbohydrate enters the bloodstream the greater insulin secretion.

Insulin is an anabolic hormone. As such, it is also responsible for the growth of adipose tissue (fat gain) through an increased conversion of carbohydrates into fat.

Thus, the lower the glycemic index of a food, the lower insulin secretion and the less likely the tendency of a carbohydrate to be converted to fat.

Furthermore, the low-GI foods have been shown to cause a longer lasting feeling of satiety after a meal that blunts the tendency crave sugar between meals!

Low GI foods reduce calorie intake at the next meal. This is an important aspect, since it will enable you to successfully stick to a calorie restricted diet for long periods of time without starving!

Instead, foods with high glycemic index (eg white bread, white pasta, white rice, puffed rice cakes, corn, carrots, etc.) are responsible for a feeling of fullness and less excessive food intake at the next meal.

These are the main reasons why people with high intake of foods glycemic index, while on a calorie restriction diet can not stick to it for long periods of time and therefore fail to lose fat permanently. Change your dietary sources of carbohydrates for low-GI foods if you want to be successful in your goal to lose stomach fat and weight quicker.

29. Limit consumption of fructose

Fructose is a simple sugar that is contained in fruits.

It is a controversial type of sugar - once being a simple sugar that I think goes into the bloodstream at a faster rate and therefore should lead to greater insulin secretion, which would ultimately promote fat gain.

30. High Intensity Weight Training to lose stomach fat and weight

Intensity is a measure of physical effort given by:

Number of repetitions.
Weight used.
Rest period between sets.
Manipulating each factor intensity varies.

High intensity resistance training results in fat loss ideal for two main aspects:

1. High intensity increases levels of "adrenaline" and "Noradrenaline". Adrenaline and noradrenaline are hormones. These two hormones target specific receptors located

69

on fat cells that are responsible for fat loss.

2. The high intensity weight training promotes the production of a high amount of lactic acid. Research has shown that lactic acid enhances the secretion of growth hormone (GH). Growth Hormone is also one of the most powerful agents of fat loss.

Thus, increasing the intensity of workouts you will lose stomach fat and weight.

Part 2: Emotional Eating

Tackling Emotional Eating

When eating becomes an alternative to trying to cover an emotional void, you must be alert.

Who has not had an inexplicable desire to eat something just for greed? Used it to reduce anxiety or take care of our PMS or eat after fighting with partners or simply pressures at work. Food is a quick and unhealthy way to deal with problems.

First of all, we need to understand what compulsion is and how it works. Usually it appears when something is wrong (difficulty in relationships with parents, loss, separation, etc.) and puts in a huge void within us. As this feeling of emptiness is too bad, our unconscious ends up finding a way to ease our pain, whether from food, drink, sex, shopping, drugs, etc..

The problem is that the gap persists and requires more, i.e. the person ends up becoming a compulsive in the attempt to "cover" this "emotional hole." Unfortunately for such an emotional issue the only solution is to find the cause and deal with it which can often be difficult and painful. Eating a box of chocolates for breakfast is a more enjoyable task.

Overcoming Abdominal Fat by Carmen Beese

So why the choice of food? Our first experience of love is through breastfeeding. In addition to breast milk to satisfy our hunger, the maternal lap provides the feeling of comfort and safety and therefore, from birth we learn to associate food with the "warmth".

So what to do to combat emotional eating?

Usually the person who suffers from compulsive eating is a little anxious and wants quick solutions. After all there is that "aching void", which makes the individual look for miracle diets, medications and even surgery to reduce the stomach.

Even the stomach reduction surgery without nutritional and psychological follow-up can be a disaster. There is one case I once read in a medical report where after surgery this lady had failed to lose the desired weight, as her hunger was uncontrollable and she ate dozens of mashed bananas with condensed milk for two days. The creamy paste which formed was easier to digest than normal solid food therefore she was able to continue eating uncontrollably.

The stories are numerous. So do not even try for quick solutions to lose belly fat without treating your emotional eating first. A good example is people who quit smoking more often get fat. Simply put the compulsion was substituted from cigarettes to food.

As hard as it is to face your problem of emotional eating, nothing is more rewarding than caring for and healing the wounds of the past and being able to move on, without the void inside, without regret and without guilt.

Think about it, the choice to be happy is in your hands.

Night Eating Disorder

Anguish and anxiety can precipitate a night eating disorder responsible for night raids to the fridge.

Some prefer to close their mouths before going to sleep; others prefer to eat a light meal. But there are still those who do not dismiss a good meal and a dessert. In some cases, the habit can be a disorder that must be addressed. The people who suffer from this usually eat very little during the day and raid the fridge at night. Distress and anxiety are all factors that can precipitate an eating disorder at night.

When the desire to eat comes, the person feels the need to eat anything as a way to relieve stress or emotional needs.

How to treat

73

Now you have discovered the night eating disorder, it's time to treat it. Cognitive therapy and behavioral therapy are the most suitable, in some cases, it is recommended the use of antidepressants and sleep regulators, especially when there is a decline in mood.

A good tip on how to control the night eating disorder is changing food for things that give pleasure. A good shower or bath, going out and exercising can help. However, if the crisis hits and it is hard to resist, make the fridge your ally. Keep the right food in there!

The trick is to eat a balanced diet in all meals. Ideally, all nutrients like carbohydrates, proteins, lipids, vitamins and minerals are balanced according to the needs of the person.

As the metabolism slows down at night, it is preferable to consume fruits, wholegrain (brown bread, brown rice, whole grains), lean protein (chicken breast and white fish), skimmed yogurt, vegetables and teas. The most suitable fruit are apple, papaya, pear, pineapple, grape and strawberry.

The meal must have a good variety of vegetables, at least four different colors. Fatty foods, white breads, white rice, biscuits, fried food and sweets and deserts should be off the menu at night.

A poor diet also affects the quality of sleep. Alcoholic beverages and foods containing

74

caffeine such as some kinds of tea and chocolate, are stimulants and can interfere with sleep. As far as time is concerned, experts recommend that you wait at least 3 hours before you go to bed after dinner. However, light snacks are fine.

Part 3: Metabolism

What is Metabolism?

Some people think that the metabolism is a kind of organ, or a body part, that influences digestion.

Actually, the metabolism isn't any particular body part.

It's the *process* by which the body converts food into energy.

Hence, you've likely heard of the phrase *metabolic process* used synonymously with the term *metabolism*, because they both mean the same thing.

The Medical Mumbo Jumbo

This isn't a complicated medical text (which should be great news to most of you!), and so we don't need to spend an unnecessary amount of time and space focusing on the layered complexity of the human body and its extraordinary intelligence.

Overcoming Abdominal Fat by Carmen Beese

Yet without drilling deeply into medical details -- which are not relevant for our general understanding purposes -- it's helpful to briefly look at the biological mechanisms behind metabolism.

Metabolism, as mentioned above, is the process of transforming food (e.g. nutrients) into fuel (e.g. energy). The body uses this energy to conduct a vast array of essential functions.

In fact, your ability to read this page – literally – is driven by your metabolism.

If you had *no* metabolism – that is, if you had no metabolic process that was converting food into energy – then you wouldn't be able to move.

In fact, long before you realized that you couldn't move a finger or lift your foot, your internal processes would have stopped; because the basic building blocks of life – circulating blood, transforming oxygen into carbon dioxide, expelling potentially lethal

Overcoming Abdominal Fat by Carmen Beese

wastes through the kidneys and so on – *all of these* depend on metabolism.

Keep this in mind the next time you hear someone say that they have a *slow metabolism*.

While they may struggle with unwanted weight gain due to metabolic factors, they certainly have a *functioning metabolism*.

If they didn't, they wouldn't even be able to speak (because that, too, requires energy that comes from, you guessed it: metabolism!).

It's also interesting to note that, while we conveniently refer to the *metabolic process* as if it were a single function, it's really a catch-all term for countless functions that are taking place inside the body. Every second of every minute of every day of your life – even, of course, when you sleep – numerous chemical conversions are taking place through metabolism, or metabolic functioning.

Overcoming Abdominal Fat by Carmen Beese

In a certain light, the metabolism has been referred to as a harmonizing process that manages to achieve two critical bodily functions that, in a sense, seem to be at odds with each other.

Anabolism and Catabolism

The first function is creating tissue and cells. Each moment, our bodies are creating more cells to replace dead or dysfunctional cells.

For example, if you cut your finger, your body (if it's functioning properly) will begin – without even wasting a moment or asking your permission –the process of creating skin cells to clot the blood and start the healing process. This creation process is indeed a metabolic response, and is called *anabolism*.

On the other hand, there is the exact *opposite* activity taking place in other parts of the body. Instead of building cells and tissue through metabolism, the body is breaking down energy so that the body can do what it's supposed to do.

For example, as you aerobically exercise, your body temperature rises as your heart beat increases and remains with a certain range.

As this happens, your body requires more oxygen; and as such, your breathing increases as you intake more H_2O. All of this, as you can imagine, requires additional energy.

After all, if your body couldn't adjust to this enhanced requirement for oxygen (both taking it in and getting rid of it in the form of carbon dioxide), you would collapse!

Presuming, of course, that you *aren't* overdoing it, your body will instead begin converting food (e.g. calories) into energy. And this process, as you know, is a metabolic process, and is called *catabolism*.

So as you can see, the metabolism is a *constant* process that takes care of two seemingly opposite function: anabolism that uses energy to *create* cells, and catabolism that *breaks down* cells to create energy.

Indeed, it's in this way that the metabolism earns its reputation as a harmonizer. It

Overcoming Abdominal Fat by Carmen Beese

brings together these apparently conflicting functions, and does so in an optimal way that enables the body to create cells as needed, and break them down, again as needed.

Metabolism and Weight Loss

By now, you already have a sense of how metabolism relates to weight loss (catabolic metabolism, or breaking cells down and transforming them into energy).

To understand this process even more clearly, we can introduce a very important player in the weight loss game: the *calorie*.

Calories

Calories are simply units of measure. They aren't actually *things* in and of themselves; they are labels for other things, just like how an inch really isn't anything, but it measures the distance between two points.

So what do calories measure?

Easy: they measure *energy*.

Yup, the evil calorie – the bane of the dieter's existence – is really just a 3-syllable label for energy.

And it's important to highlight this, because the body itself, despite its vast intelligence (much of which medical science cannot yet understand, only appreciate in awe) does not really do a very intelligent job of distinguishing good energy from bad.

Actually, to be blunt, the body doesn't *care* about where the energy comes from. Let's explore this a little more, because it's very important to the overall understanding of how to boost your metabolism, particularly when we look at food choices.

In our choice-laden grocery stores, with dozens of varieties of foods – hundreds, perhaps – there seems to be a fairly clear awareness of what's *good* food, and what's *bad* or *junk* food.

For example, we don't need a book to remind us that, all else being equal, a plum is a *good* food, whereas a tub of thick and

82

creamy double-fudge ice cream is a *bad* food.

Not bad tasting, of course; but, really, you won't find many fit people eating a vat of ice cream a day, for obvious reasons. So what does this have to do with calories and energy?

It's this: while *you and I* can evaluate our food choices and say that something (like a plum) is a healthy source of energy, and something else (like a tub of ice cream) is an unhealthy source of energy, *the body doesn't evaluate*. Really.

It sounds strange and amazing, but the body really doesn't care. To the body, *energy is energy*. It takes whatever it gets, and doesn't really *know* that some foods are healthier than others. It's kind of like a garbage disposal: it takes what you put down it, whether it *should* go down or not.

So let's apply this to the body, and to weight gain. When the body receives a calorie – which, as we know, is merely a label for *energy* – it must do something with that energy.

In other words, putting all other nutrients and minerals aside, if a plum delivers 100 calories to the body, it *has* to accept those 100 calories. The same goes for 500 calories from a (small) tub of ice cream: those 500 calories *have* to be dealt with.

Now, the body does two things to that energy: it either metabolizes it via anabolism, or it metabolizes it via catabolism. That is, it will either convert the energy (calories) into cells/tissue, or it will use that energy (calories) to break down cells.

Now the link between calories/energy, metabolism, and weight loss becomes rather clear and direct.

When there is an excess of energy, and the body can't use this energy to deal with any needs at the time, **it will be forced to create cells with that extra energy.** It has to.

Overcoming Abdominal Fat by Carmen Beese

It doesn't necessarily *want* to, but after figuring out that the energy can't be used to do anything (such as help you exercise or digest some food), it *has* to turn it into cells through anabolism.

And those extra cells? Yup, you guessed it: added weight!

In a nutshell (and nuts have lots of calories by the way, so watch out and eat them in small portions...), the whole calorie/metabolism/weight gain thing is really just about excess energy.
When there are too many calories in the body – that is, when there's *too much energy* from food – then the body transforms those calories into *stuff*.

And that *stuff*, most of the time, is fat. Sometimes, of course, those extra calories are transformed into muscle; and this is usually a good thing for those watching their weight or trying to maintain an optimal body fat ratio.

In fact, because muscles require calories to maintain, people with strong muscle tone *burn calories* without actually doing anything; their metabolism burns it for them.

This is the primary reason why exercising and building lean muscle is part of an overall program to boost your metabolism; because the more lean muscle you have, the more *places* excess calories can go *before* they're turned into fat.

A Final Word About Fat

There's a nasty rumor floating around out there that fat cells are *permanent*. And the nastiest thing about this rumor is that it's true.

Yes, most experts conceded that fat cells – once created – are there for life. Yet this doesn't spell doom and gloom to those of us who could stand to *drop a few pounds*. Because even though experts believe that fat cells are permanent, they also agree that fat cells can be *shrunk*. So even if the absolute number of fat cells in your body remains the same, their size – and hence their appearance and percentage of your overall weight – can be reduced.

Recap

So while we haven't gone into any medical detail – because we don't need to or want to – we have covered some key basics about metabolism. In fact, you probably know as much about metabolism now as many so-called experts.

The bottom line is simply that metabolism represents a process – countless processes, in fact – that convert food into energy. When this process creates cells, it's called anabolism. When this process breaks cells down, it's called catabolism.

For people trying to lose weight, it's important to experience *catabolism*. That is, it's important to convert food into energy that is used to break cells down.

Catabolism is also important because it prevents excess energy (calories) from being stored by the body.

Remember: when the body has too many calories – regardless of what food source those calories came from – it can only do two things. It can desperately try and see if you have any energy needs (like maybe you're running a marathon at the time).

Or, more often, it will *have* to store those calories. It has no choice. And unless you have lean muscle that is gobbling up those excess calories, you'll be adding fat.

The remainder of this book, however, is going to point you in the *opposite* direction. You'll learn various techniques, tips, and strategies to boost your metabolism.

And then, in the latter part of this book, you'll be introduced to some metabolism-boosting foods that you'll surely want to add to your regular eating regimen.

Tips, Techniques, and Strategies for Boosting Your Metabolism

If you're reading this book, chances are that you've tried – at least *once* in your life – to boost your metabolism.

Perhaps (like most of us) you weren't quite certain what a metabolism *was*, and perhaps

Overcoming Abdominal Fat by Carmen Beese

(again, like most of us) you probably didn't quite know all that you needed to know in order to accomplish your goals.

Maybe you started a rigorous exercise program of jogging and muscle toning.

Or maybe you started eating several small portions a day, rather than three large traditional *meal-sized* portions.

Or maybe you started taking all kinds of supplements that promised to boost your metabolism.

The thing is, is that *all* of these methods can indeed work.

Really: exercise, eating strategically, and ensuring that your body has catabolism-friendly supplements are but three of many generally good ideas.

So what's the problem?

The problem is that many of us have no real scientific understanding of *what, how, or why* these methods boost metabolism.

Some of us, in fact, don't really even know if they work; we just think that they do.

For example, a person may start a vigorous exercise program that includes significant aerobic cardiovascular movement, such as jogging or cycling.

And indeed, after a week, that person may notice a drop in weight.

Yet is this due to a boosted metabolism? Maybe, maybe not! Could it be due to water loss through perspiration that hasn't been adequately replenished? Maybe, maybe not!

The point here is that many people – at risk to their health and wellness – don't quite understand the tips, strategies, and techniques of boosting their metabolism. And that's what we're going to rectify in this chapter.

In this book, you won't come across any casual information that *a friend of a friend heard on TV*. Nor will you be subjected to off-the-cuff information of how to boost your metabolism.

Rather, we're going to look at the popular, easy, fun (yes, believe it or not), and *successful* ways to boost your metabolism.

The popular and widely respected Internet publication *i-Village* highlights 11 key ways to speed up metabolism. To most easily introduce and discuss them here, we've taken these 11 key ideas and broken them down into 3 broad categories:

1. Exercise
2. Lifestyle
3. Diet

As you go through each of the 11 key points, you'll certainly note that there is some overlap between them. For example, it's hard to imagine that introducing exercise into your life isn't, in many ways, a *lifestyle* choice.

Similarly, integrating all kinds of metabolism-boosting foods into your diet is surely going to influence how you spend your time (probably less time in fast food line-ups, for one!).

So with this being said, *please* don't get bogged down in the categories; they are merely provided here to help organize these points, and to help you easily refer to them in the future. The important thing for you to do is understand each of the 11 points, and evaluate how you can responsibly integrate them into your life.

1. Exercise

It's going to be *old news* for you to be reminded that exercising is a bit part of boosting your metabolism and burning up calories.

Unless you're born with one of those *unusually active metabolisms* which allows you to, almost freakishly, eat thousands of calories a day without weight-gain consequences, you're like the vast majority of us who need to give your metabolisms a bit of a kick through exercising.

Now, you might think that cardiovascular (aerobic) exercise is an important part of boosting your metabolism; and you'd be right!

Provided that, of course, your qualified doctor confirms that you're able to start a program of cardiovascular exercise, this is indeed the place to start. Increasing heart rate, blood circulation, body temperature, and oxygen intake/carbon dioxide exchange all send messages to the system to initiate catabolism (breaking down cells and using them for energy).

Yet if cardiovascular exercising is the place to start, does that mean that it's the place to end? *No!*

Many people, who aren't as educated as you'll be when you've finished this book, responsibly start a dedicated program of cardiovascular health, but they *don't go any further.* Not because they're lazy; but because, frankly, they don't know that there is significantly *more* that they can do in their home gym, or at the fitness club, that will boost their metabolism even more potently.

We focus upon these added activities now, below.

Build Muscle

Many people – particularly some women – are very leery about undertaking any exercise regimen that can lead to muscle building.

The old perception was that muscle building leads to *muscle bulking*, and before long, gorging forearm veins and other unwanted results. This is, frankly, not the case.

Provided that women aren't supporting their workouts with specific muscle-building supplements, there is no need to be concerned; because building lean muscle won't make them *bulk up*.

Still, however, the question remains: why would women (and, of course, men) who want to boost their metabolism focus on muscle building? Isn't cardiovascular exercising the *only* thing that matters?

94

Again, the answer is: No! In *addition* to a healthy and responsible cardiovascular program, muscle building is an exceptionally powerful way to boost metabolism.

How? Because a pound of muscle burns more calories than a pound of fat.

And what does this mean? It means (and get ready to stare in awe) that if you have more muscle on your body – *anywhere on your body* – you will simply burn more calories as a result.

You don't even have to *do* anything. You'll simply burn more calories, because muscle simply requires more of an energy investment.

Of course, as you can infer, if you build muscle and then leave it alone, over time, the muscle fibers will weaken and you'll lose that wonderful calorie-burning factory. But that's no problem, because all you need to do is build and maintain healthy muscle.

It may sound daunting; especially if at the moment you perceive yourself to have much more fat than muscle.

Yet the important thing for you to remember is that once you start building muscle – through any kind of strength training – your body will *itself* start burning more calories.

It has to; even while you sleep, or go to a movie, or read a book. It's like putting your calorie-burning (catabolism) program on auto-pilot.

So don't let a little (or even a lot) of extra flab, at the moment, deter you from believing that muscle building is important.

Yes, you should enjoy cardiovascular exercise too, because that's ultimately how your body is going to burn existing fat. But muscle building plays a profoundly supportive role in that pursuit.

And it's an exponential one, too: the more fat you transform into muscle, the more calories you'll burn simply to maintain that new muscle (and the wonderful cycle goes on and on!).

Interval Training

The basic weight loss *nuts and bolts* behind cardiovascular exercise (or any kind of exercise, really) is, as you know, a matter of catabolism.

Essentially, if you can engineer your body to require more energy, your body will comply by breaking cells down to deliver it; and that process (metabolism) burns calories.
Simple, right?

So based on that logic, something called *interval training* neatly fits in with the overall plan. Interval training is simply adding a high-energy burning component to your exercise plan on an infrequent, or *interval*, basis.

For example, you may be at a stage where you can jog for 20 minutes every other day, and thus put your heart into a cardiovascular zone during this time.

This, obviously, is going to help you boost your metabolism and thus burn calories/energy. Yet you can actually burn *disproportionately more* calories if, during that 20 minute jog, you add a 30 second or 1 minute sprint.

Why? Because during this 30 seconds or 1 minute, you give your body a bit of a jolt.

Not an unhealthy jolt; remember, we're talking about quick bursts here, not suddenly racing around the track or through the park! By giving your body an *interval* jolt, it automatically – and somewhat unexpectedly – has to turn things up a notch.

And to compensate for your extra energy requirements, the body will burn more calories.

It's essential for you to always keep in mind that interval training *only works when it's at intervals*. This may seem like a strange thing to say (and even difficult to understand), but it's actually very straightforward.

Overcoming Abdominal Fat by Carmen Beese

The metabolism-boosting benefits that you enjoy as a result of interval training are primarily due to the fact that your body, suddenly, needs to find more energy. While it was chugging along and supplying your energy needs during your cardiovascular exercising, it all of a sudden needs to go grab some more for 30 seconds or a minute; and in *that* period, it will boost your metabolism as if it were given a nice, healthy jolt.

As you can see, if you suddenly decided to extend your 30 second or 1 minute sprint into a *20 minute sprint*, you simply wouldn't experience all of the benefits.

Yes, your body would use more energy if you extend yourself to the higher range of your aerobic training zone. But your body won't necessarily get that *jolt* that only comes from interval training.

So remember: your goal with interval training is to give your body a *healthy jolt* where it suddenly says to itself:

Overcoming Abdominal Fat by Carmen Beese

"Whoa! We need more energy here FAST, this person has increased their heart rate from 180 beats per minute to 190 beats per minute! Let's go to any available cell, like those fat cells down at the waist, and break them down via catabolism so that this person can get the energy that they need!"

Remember (sorry to be repetitive, but this is very important): the whole point of interval training in this way is to give your body a sudden, limited, healthy jolt where it needs more energy – quick!

If you simply increase your speed and stay there, while your body may, overall burn some more calories, it won't get that jolt.

Also bear in mind that interval training can indeed last longer than 30 seconds or a minute.

Some experts suggest that you can use interval training for 30-40 *minutes*,

Overcoming Abdominal Fat by Carmen Beese

depending on your state of health and what your overall exercise regimen looks like.

The reason we're focusing on 30 seconds to 1 minute is simply to give you a clear understanding that interval training is a kind of mini *training within a training* program.

And, as always, *don't* overdo it with your interval training. Your goal here is to become healthier and stronger, and lose weight in that process.

You gain nothing if you run so fast or bike so hard during interval training that you hurt yourself. You will actually undermine your own health, and possibly have to stop exercising while torn muscles or other ailments heal.

Variety

They say that variety is the spice of life, and this is indeed quite true. But despite this awareness, many people don't *spice up* their exercise program; which is surprising, since doing so often leads to valuable metabolism-boosting benefits.

There are a few easy ways to add variety to your exercise program. We've already talked about interval training, and that is indeed one way to shift your body's *metabolic engine* into a higher gear.

Other effective ways are to break up a longer routine into smaller parts.

For example, instead of committing to 1x1 hour workout a day, it can be metabolism-boosting to split this up into 2x30 minute workouts; or even, on some occasions, 3x20 minute workouts.

Furthermore, you can add variety into your daily exercise routine without formally *exercising*.

For example, you can take the stairs instead of the elevator. Or you can start your day with a brisk walk instead of a coffee and the newspaper.

Or, instead of parking close to the grocery store entrance, you can walk the distance between a far away parking spot and the entrance.

All of these tips provide two metabolism-boosting benefits.

Firstly, as you can easily see, they can make exercising more *fun*. While, indeed, it's important to have an exercise routine, you don't want to have a *boring* exercise routine (because then your chances of stopping are that much great!).

So adding these new elements to your overall exercise commitment simply helps encourage you to stick with the program. And since exercising is a core part of boosting your metabolism, any technique or tip that helps you continue exercising over the long term is a wise piece of advice.

The second important benefit of variety in your exercise program leads us back to the interval training concept, discussed above.

When you add variety to your workout, your body cannot get into a *groove*. Remember: the body is a remarkable piece of work, and will always strive to do things efficiently.

Overcoming Abdominal Fat by Carmen Beese

Naturally, the overall state of your health (which can be influenced by genetics and other factors outside of your control) will play a role in *how* efficiently your body runs.

But regardless of how your body is put together and what genetic influences you have to deal with, your body really likes you, and wants to do things *as efficiently as it possibly can.*

Therefore, when you start exercising, your body can start to develop a kind of expectation of energy output. It's not doing this to be lazy; it's doing this because, quite sincerely, it wants to help!

If your body starts to *predict* that you need a certain amount of energy to complete a certain task (such as jog for 20 minutes), then it will start to achieve that energy output more efficiently.

For example, when you first start jogging for, say, 2 minutes a time followed by 5 minutes of walking, your body may require a great deal of energy to help you achieve this.

And as a result, you may find yourself very out of breath or tired as your body strives to meet this increased demand. Naturally, of course, *catabolism* will be involved, and your body metabolism will increase.

But over time, say a month or so, your body will simply become more efficient. It will have become stronger, and will be able to supply your energy needs much more efficiently; you may not even break a sweat!

What's happened here is that your health has improved; your body has to *work less hard* to provide you with your energy needs.

Ironically, this can actually obscure your metabolism-boosting efforts; because, as you know, you want to tell your body to start the catabolism process. But if your body is efficiently working, it won't really dig into its reserves (e.g. fat cells) in order to provide you with the energy that you need.

So the trick is to keep *variety* in your workouts. Many people choose to cross-train for this very reason. It not only targets different muscle groups, but it keeps your

105

body from finding a *groove* whereby it tried to help you by slowing down metabolism.

Remember: your body doesn't read books like this; it doesn't need to, and it doesn't *care*.

It has no *clue* that a speedier metabolism is *"good"* or "*bad"*. Now, as far as you and I are concerned, we know that a speedy metabolism is a *good thing* in our weight loss efforts.

But your body doesn't make this evaluation. And so it won't turn on its metabolism jets because you want it to.

You can't (unfortunately) send a memo to your body and ask it to *please speed up metabolism.*

If you *could*, then that would be amazing! But that's not reality at all. What we have to do is *force* the body to say to itself: *hey, I need to speed up metabolism because this person needs more energy!*

And one of the best ways for you to *force* the body to have this kind of thinking is to add variety to your workouts.

2. Lifestyle

When we come across the term *lifestyle*, we tend to think of the basic day-to-day habits that we rely on; sometimes without giving them much of a second thought. And this is indeed the case when we talk about how lifestyle influences the speed of your metabolism.

Now, quite honestly, most of us live busy lives in one form or another, and therefore it's challenging to really keep an eye on *all* of our habits.

Balancing work, family, hobbies, and other commitments often means that our lifestyle isn't so much of a *choice*, as it is a necessity.

Yet with respect to the fact that many of us face sincere limitations in our *lifestyle choices*, there are many things that we can do – little things, but important things – that can help speed up our metabolism.

107

So if you're a bit put-off by the term *lifestyle*, please don't skim over this section. The little things that you change in your regular, day-to-day lifestyle can indeed have the most profound influence on the speed of your metabolism, and the achievement of your short and long-term weight loss goals.

Get on the Wagon

Do you know people who carefully choose low-fat, low-calorie meal choices, are very disciplined when it comes to *not* ordering the Chef's Special pecan pie for desert, yet order a glass or two of wine with their meal?

Well, unfortunately, these people are *really* undermining their efforts to boost metabolism.

Studies show that drinking alcohol with meals actually encourages *over eating*; which means more calories that need to be burned away (or transformed into fat!).

Furthermore, many people are simply unaware that many alcoholic drinks are

108

laden with calories; almost as much as sugary-rich soft drinks.

 A bottle of beer can deliver a few hundred calories, and most cocktails are in the same range. Wine is generally considered to deliver the *least* amount of calories; but even this is a bit of a slippery slope.

Three glasses of wine can be worth 300 calories that the body simply has to *deal* with in one form or another.

The tip here isn't to stop drinking alcohol altogether (despite the title of this section). If you enjoy alcohol then there's no particular reason why you have to quit cold turkey, but you will save a bit of money and not consume as many calories.

Simply, the call here is that you become *aware* that it influences your metabolism. If you consume excess alcohol (even without becoming inebriated), you force your system to deal with more calories.

And unless you're compensating for these added calories through exercise or muscle

Overcoming Abdominal Fat by Carmen Beese

building, catabolism cannot occur. Instead, anabolism will inevitably occur, and new cells will be created from those calories (mostly fat cells).

Sleep

This is a toughie. Most of us don't have as much control over the amount that we sleep as we *should*. Work, family, education, housekeeping, and so many other tasks can literally prevent us from getting the amount of sleep that we need.

However, as the experts tell us, getting enough sleep actually improves metabolism. On the other hand, people who are constantly sleep deprived typically find that they have less energy to do regular, daily activities; including *digestion*.

As a result, sleep-starved people often lower their own metabolism. They simply don't have the strength to break down food efficiently, particularly carbohydrates.

This is a very difficult issue, because many people can only find time to exercise by *borrowing from* their rest time.

For example, after a long day of work and dealing with family and home commitments, a person may find that the only time they have to exercise (and thus boost their metabolism) is late at night; say around 9:00 pm, or even later. So what should one do?

Ultimately, it's a question of balance. Naturally, if you're willing to exercise, and your doctor agrees that it's healthy for you to do that, then you're *not* going to get fit by sleeping instead of exercising.

Yet with that being said, if you steal time away from your sleep/rest in order to exercise, over time, you can actually do more harm than good; because the following day, you won't have enough energy to digest what you eat. The answer to this catch-22 lies in *balance*.

You don't have to work out every night. Or perhaps you can integrate a workout into your life during the day; maybe at lunchtime or right after work.

Most fitness clubs are open very early (some are even open 24 hours), and if you choose to workout at home, you can do so in a generally affordable way (while some machines can cost thousands, basic machines that get the job done only cost a few hundred, even cheaper if they're used).

If you find that you have trouble sleeping, then this can also negatively affect the speed of your metabolism (because you won't have enough energy the following day). Insomnia and other sleep disorders are *very common problems*, and there exists a variety of support systems in place to help people get the rest that they require. Some non-medical tips to help you fall asleep include:

- ✓ Don't eat late at night
- ✓ Try drinking warm milk before bedtime
- ✓ Don't turn on the TV at night
- ✓ Try yoga or other stress-relieving practices

✓ Try having a warm bath before bedtime
✓ Don't exercise close to bedtime; your body can become so energized that it doesn't want to sleep!

Relax

We briefly noted *yoga* in the list above of *Things to Do*, and that brings us to another key influence of your metabolism: stress.

Believe it or not, but experts are now telling us that stress can send unwanted signals to our body; signals that lead to slower metabolism.

Essentially, what happens is that when the body is under constant stress, it releases *stress hormones* that flood the system.

These stress-related hormones actually tell the body to create larger fat cells in the abdomen. The result can be both increased weight (through increased fat cells), and a slower metabolism.

Obviously, these are *two very negative factors* in the quest to boost metabolism and lose weight. The last thing that we want is more and *bigger* fat cells in our abdomen, coupled with a diminished metabolism!

Yet this is, tragically, what happens to many people who experience constant, continuous stress. And, alas, this is *many people*; especially those of us who have to balance so many competing objectives, such as work, family, and other vital tasks.

So the advice here is indeed to "relax and chill out", and there are some simple techniques that can, and should, be added to your life.

These include walking more, listening to relaxing music, meditation, yoga, eating non-stimulating foods (e.g. no caffeine, no sugar, and so on), and building a daily regimen that includes periodic *time outs* where you can re-center yourself and de-stress.

Remember: while relaxing is good advice for anyone, it's important for you to note that stress *negatively influences metabolism*. So there is a link between how much stress you experience and your ability to break down cells and lose weight.

So if you don't want to *relax* because you don't have the time, then you should realize that your stressed-out life is probably playing a role in your weight gain/your inability to lose weight.

There's Something GOOD About This Time of the Month!?

Now here's a strange one that is *for the ladies,* only.

Studies have demonstrated that the 2-week period prior to the onset of PMS is one in which fat burning capacity is at a premium.

This is ironic indeed; because that's usually the period in which women *don't* want to workout; because their body and its emotional computer are preparing for PMS. However, studies in Australia have shown that women were able to burn off as much as 30% more fat in the 2 weeks preceding PMS.

Overcoming Abdominal Fat by Carmen Beese

The reason for this, researchers argue, is because this is when the female body's production of estrogen and progesterone are at their highest.

Since these hormones tell the body to use fat as a source of energy, exercising during this time can really pay off. The body will be inclined to target fat cells for catabolism.

3. Diet

Ah yes, diet. For most of us, our information concerning metabolism is related in one way or another to eating. Most of us have been told of metabolism-friendly foods, or metabolism *unfriendly* foods.

But really, while we may be basically aware that, all else being equal, a stalk of celery is better for your metabolism than fries with gravy, our understanding of diet and metabolism is pretty low.

To fix this, the following section looks at some powerful and scientific diet-related tips that will boost your metabolism. Indeed, as you'll soon learn, it's not merely what you eat that matters; it's when, and how, too.

Don't Hate Calories

The word calorie has a bad rap. We constantly come across *calorie reduced* or *low calorie* foods. And it's not uncommon to overhear someone gasp about the immense *calorie content* of certain foods, such as a rich and creamy desert, or a giant fast food burger.

All of this anti-calorie rhetoric therefore has made a lot of us pretty calorie-*phobic*; as soon as we see something that has lots of them, we run away. But is this wise?

Yes and no. Yes, it's wise in the sense that avoiding that double-layer chocolate fudge cake for desert is probably a good idea (actually, scratch that; it *is* a good idea).

The calories that come from the cake are really going to be the so-called *empty calorie* kind; which means that there's no real nutritional value that your body can squeeze out and make use of.

117

But in the bigger picture, it's *unwise* for your metabolism to become calorie-avoidant.

Why? Because your body is a marvellous machine that tries, at all times, to do what it can to make your life easier.

Indeed, while it may not always function at optimal levels (for a variety of reasons, including genetics), it still tries to do its very best. The body, for all of its limitations and so forth, is *not* a lazy thing!

With this in mind, the body is always trying to keep itself alive and functioning in the manner that it deems to be healthiest.

And that's why if you suddenly decrease the amount of calories that you need, your body won't try to *do more with less*. In other words, your body won't respond in the way that you want it to: it won't necessarily provoke catabolism and thus reduce weight and fat cells.

Instead, your smart and wise body will try to *keep you alive* by slowing down its metabolism. It will simply believe that something is wrong – maybe you're trapped somewhere without food – and it will just begin to become very stingy with energy.

So what's the end result? If your body needs 2000 calories a day to survive, and you suddenly give it only 1000, it *won't* begin to burn off 1000 calories worth of cells that you have lying around on your love handles.

Instead, your body will *slow down its metabolism*. It will really try and get as much energy out of those 1000 calories, because it doesn't want to waste anything.

Physically, you'll naturally feel more tired because your body is being very miserly with energy, and will devote its 1000-calorie ration to essential systems, like blood and oxygen supply (and others).

Metabolically, you won't be burning off extra calories. In fact, you can actually *gain weight* by dramatically reducing your calorie intake!

The flipside of this, of course, is that you should consume a daily caloric intake that is proportionate to your body size, type, and weight loss goals.

And then, once you determine the amount of calories that you need (probably with the aid of a qualified nutritionist or fitness expert); you can provide that to your body via healthy, efficient calories.

For example, if your body needs 1500 calories per day, and one slice of double-fudge chocolate cake delivers a whopping 500 of those, then you can see that eating just one of these slices will take up a full 1/3rd of your daily caloric needs; and that's not good!

On the other hand, you can see that drinking a tasty fruit smoothy made with yogurt and nuts can deliver half as many calories, but provide you with essential nutrients, vitamins, and other elements that your body needs to healthily do its work.

Eat More?

Fresh on the heels of the discussion on calories, it's also helpful to note that eating frequently throughout the day can be very good for boosting metabolism. There are a couple of reasons for this.

The first reason is that people who tend to eat throughout the day do considerably less *snacking*. As a result, they tend to avoid the potato chips or candy bars that they might otherwise consume if they suddenly felt *hungry*.

People who eat throughout the day don't tend to experience severe *hunger pangs*, because they don't reach that stage.

The second reason, and the one that you can probably guess based on your understanding of metabolism, is that by eating throughout the day, you are constantly keeping your metabolism in motion.

It's kind of like having a generator run all the time; it will simply use more electricity than if you powered it on 3 times a day.

Overcoming Abdominal Fat by Carmen Beese

Now, it goes without saying (but we should say it anyway just in case!) that just because it's *good* for metabolism-boosting to eat frequently, this *doesn't* mean that you can eat *junk* all day long!

Rather, if you choose to eat more frequently, then you'll certainly need to be very aware of *what* you eat; because you can easily exceed your required amount of daily calories if you don't keep an eye on this.

That's why, if your plan is to follow the eat-more-to-burn-more approach, then you should keep a food journal that notes what you eat (and drink of course) throughout the day.

You should not merely know the calorie levels of what you eat, but you should know the overall nutritional values, too.

For example, if you're on target to eat 50 grams of protein per day, then you want to make sure you reach this target and not exceed it (or come in below it).

In other words, merely focusing on calories is only half of the job. You will need to ensure that you're eating enough protein, carbohydrates, fats (the good unsaturated kind!), and the other vitamins and minerals that your body needs in order to function at optimal levels.

Eat Early

We've all heard that *breakfast is the most important meal of the day*. And in terms of boosting your metabolism, this is indeed the case! There are a couple of reasons why eating a hearty and healthy breakfast can boost metabolism and lead to weight loss goals.

The first reason is that people who eat breakfast are much less inclined to snack throughout the morning. For example, if you had a good breakfast of fruit and low-sugar cereal in the morning, your chances of visiting the vending machine at work around 10:30am diminish significantly.

Of course, as you recall from our previous discussion on eating more frequently, this doesn't mean that you shouldn't eat something between breakfast and lunch.

Overcoming Abdominal Fat by Carmen Beese

It simply means that, since you won't be extremely hungry at 10:30am (because you skipped breakfast), you'll be less inclined to eat *anything* that you get your hands on; such as a nice donut that your co-worker was kind enough to offer you.

In other words, by starting your day in a nutritious way, you'll have more control over *what* you eat throughout the day.

The second reason is more aligned with metabolism-boosting. Studies have shown that metabolism slows during sleep, and doesn't typically get going again until you eat.

Therefore, starting the day with breakfast is like kick-starting your metabolism. You'll actually burn more calories throughout the day, simply by eating breakfast (hey, who knew?!).

Remember: as you eat your breakfast, control both the portion and the contents. You don't want to eat to the point of complete fullness; because, remember, you want to eat throughout the day and you won't be able to do that if you're *stuffed*.

At the same time, beware of high-fat breakfasts. Studies have shown that high-fat breakfasts, such as those that include bacon and sausage, not only deliver *lots of calories* (there are 9 calories for every gram of fat, as compared to 4 for every gram of carbohydrates and proteins, respectively).

But they also can make you very hungry again, very soon! So in addition to having ingested a lot of fat (and hence a lot of calories), you'll typically find yourself rather ravenous again in a few hours.

Alternatively, breakfasts that are high in fiber take longer to digest, and thus, the body won't be hungry again for a while.

This is something to bear in mind; and it may explain why many people who eat breakfast find themselves *painfully hungry* by lunchtime; it's not their "overactive metabolism" at work; it's the high fat content, which has been swiftly digested.

Overcoming Abdominal Fat by Carmen Beese

Befriend Protein and Good Carbs

There is a *dizzying* array of things that you can eat these days. Truly, a trip to the grocery store can be an adventure. Everywhere you turn, there's yet another food promising you *healthy this* or *weight loss that*.

Added to this confusion is that there are some foods that are beneficial for metabolic boosting, and some that *aren't*; and the differences aren't always well-known. Fortunately, we're going to tackle this problem right now and describe the three basic food groups/types that are indeed good for a speedy metabolism.

In terms of protein, studies have shown that having enough protein in your system can actually increase the speed of your metabolism. This is because protein is difficult to break down. Or rather, it *requires more energy* to break down. It's like feeding the body a knot; it needs a bit of time to unravel it.

And, as you know, when your body spends time on something, it *spends energy* (calories). And so the more time it can spend breaking down protein, the more calories that it uses.

Different people will require different amounts of protein on a daily basis. Those who exercise and build muscle will typically need more than the average amount, too.

The USFDA Food Guide suggests around 50 grams of protein a day for a *reasonably active adult*.

Keep in mind (not that you don't already have *enough* to remember, but...) that there are different sources of protein: some lean, and some high in fat. Fast food burgers may deliver up to 20 grams of protein (sometimes more), but they also deliver a great deal of *fat*; which makes them almost nutritionally worthless.

The benefits you enjoy from the protein are far outweighed by the immense fat intake; which, for some fast food burgers, can exceed 40 grams! And that's *not* including the fries (we won't even go there!).

So the thing to do is ensure that your source of protein derives from *lean* protein. Typically, protein from *some* fish and chicken is lean; though not all of it.

If you're a vegetarian, or simply looking for non-meat lean protein alternatives, low-fat cheese, legumes (lentils), and yogurt are all good sources. Simply check the food labels to determine if the source of protein is lean (doesn't deliver high fat content), or fatty.

In terms of carbohydrates, there probably isn't a more battered around micronutrient than this. It's gone from being the greatest thing in weight loss history, to one of the most reviled.
And really, it's not the fault of the innocent carbohydrate! It's really just a matter of information and knowledge, instead of speculation.

The thing to remember is that when carbohydrates are refined, such as white bread and potatoes, they are what the

Overcoming Abdominal Fat by Carmen Beese

diabetic world refers to as *high glycemic index (GI) foods*, because they require spikes in insulin in order to be digested.

As you may know, when insulin is released into the system, it promotes the storage of fat; and some experts believe that it also pushes down metabolic speed (which makes sense).

Therefore, the *good* kinds of carbohydrate to consume are those that are high in fiber, and those from fruit and vegetable sources.

Why? Because these sources of carbohydrates don't score high on the glycemic index. In other words, they don't cause a spike in insulin levels, and therefore, they don't promote fat storage.

Conclusion

We've come a long way! We now actually know more about the metabolism, and how to increase metabolic speed, than most people; and we're therefore in a position to put that information to *good use*.

We've learned that the metabolism is a process and not an actual body part.

It harmonizes two essential bodily functions: converting food into cells/tissues, and breaking cells down to provide energy. We learned that the former process is known as *anabolism*, and the latter is *catabolism*.

Indeed, it's this latter process that influences our ability to lose weight, and to keep it from coming back!

Yet going beyond the biological basics, we also learned of 3 integrated aspects of speeding up metabolism and losing weight.

These aspects were categorized in terms of: *exercise, lifestyle, and diet*. And within each of these 3 categories were a total of 11 important, practical, and quite easy ways to boost metabolism.

Now, indeed, it's the time for *action*; for as they say, wisdom is the result of experience, not study! Obviously, of course, it was essential for us to understand this subject and how it relates to boosting metabolism. So in that light, study is invaluable. But now you're equipped with the knowledge that you need.

The next step – boosting your metabolism – is all up to you.   Good luck, have fun, and enjoy your better, *leaner* healthier life!

A Final Word: Common Metabolism-Boosting Myths

The fitness experts were consulted to find the 4 most prevalent myths concerning metabolism and metabolism-boosting.

Since this book is all about reality and *not* myths, we didn't cover any of them in the actual book.   Yet, considering how common these myths are, it can indeed be useful for you to know them; and to *know* that they're myths.

That way, if you come across them in a magazine, at a fitness club, or just from the well-intentioned but misguided advice of a friend, you can confidently say (or at least just *think*): sorry, but that's a myth; I'm not going to fall for that one!

Overcoming Abdominal Fat by Carmen Beese

Myth #1: Diet Pills

The general consensus on diet pills are contained in two powerful words: BUYER BEWARE.

The problem here is that many makers of diet pills offer claims that simply aren't realistic; and if you read the fine-print of most of these advertisements, you'll see that they're really too good to be true. Little notes like *the claims made in this advertisement are not typical* should be enough of a wake-up call to realize that there's more to the story.

In some cases, diet pills can help *boost* metabolism temporarily. This, however, can be risky and generally shouldn't be done without a doctor's say-so. Unfortunately, people can become somewhat addicted to diet pills, and this can lead to disaster.

And before we go onto myth #2, remember that some diet pills are *water loss pills*. That is, they are diuretics that promote water loss, usually through excess urination. The jury on water-loss diet pills is somewhat less

open-minded than diet pills in general: THEY
DON'T WORK!

Seriously: water loss diet pills are built on
the premise that you'll lose weight through
water. And, yes, that's true: if you urinate
15 times a day, you're physically going to
weigh less.

But this is *not* actual weight loss! This is
merely unhealthy temporary weight loss, and
it will come roaring back the minute that
water stores are replenished through diet.

Or, even harder to comprehend, if a person
taking these water pills fails to restore their
body's fluid needs, they can actually suffer
dehydration; which can, and has, led to
coma and death.

Myth #2: Drop Caloric Intake

As we discussed earlier in this book (but it's
so important that it deserves an encore here
at the end), trying to lose stomach fat by
drastically cutting down calories *doesn't
work*; in fact, it's unhealthy.

The thing to remember is that the body's ability to lose weight is not controlled by calories. Calories are the input. The real control mechanism is that famous concept that you've become very familiar with: *metabolism*.

Calories are merely units of energy. It's how your body *deals* with that energy that determines whether weight is gained or lost.

So with that being said, cutting down your caloric intake to, say, 1000 calories a day isn't necessarily going to help you lose weight; because *it doesn't necessarily change your metabolism*.

Indeed, as you know, if you slow down your caloric intake, your body – which is always trying to help you in the best way that it knows how – *will slow down its metabolism*.

Really, it makes sense: the body says that something has gone wrong; instead of the 2000 calories that it needs, it's only getting 1000. The body doesn't know *why* this is happening; it doesn't know that you want to lose weight.

Overcoming Abdominal Fat by Carmen Beese

It just senses that something is wrong; perhaps you're trapped in a cave or something, or stuck in a snowstorm. So the body, trying to help you, will slow down its metabolism; it will do its best to slow down the conversion rate, so that you have as much energy *on hand* as possible.

Now, if your body was able to read this book and you could say: look, please just do what you normally do, but do it with 1000 fewer calories a day for a while, then we might actually get somewhere.

But the body doesn't work that way. It *won't* help you lose weight if you dramatically cut down on calories.

It will slow down metabolism, and (here's the worst part), if and when you ever increase calories again, your body will have to deal with that *via a slower metabolic engine*. So you can actually *gain weight* if, after cutting down your calories for a period of time, you find that you consume extra calories (say while on vacation or something).

135

Myth #3: Low Intensity Workouts

It's fair to say that *any* exercise is better than *no* exercise. So if you lead a sedentary lifestyle, then even walking around your block for 10 minutes a day is going to something positive for your body and its metabolism.

True, that difference may be imperceptible to the naked eye (or it may not?), the bottom line is that exercise is good.

Yet with this being said, some people believe that they should perform low-intensity workouts *even when* they could be performing more high-intensity workouts.

That is, instead of jogging for 20 minutes with their heart at the top end of their aerobic zone, they opt for low-intensity jogs that barely break a sweat.

Low intensity workouts simply don't lead to a faster metabolism; they *can't*. Remember, as we discussed very early in this book, metabolism is a *process*.

And that process is really one of two types: taking energy and making cells (*anabolism*), or breaking cells down to make energy (*catabolism*).

If you don't achieve a high-intensity workout, your body can't achieve catabolism; it won't need to. And the only way your body is going to go and break down existing cells is if it *needs to*.

So keep this in mind as you exercise, either at home or at a gym. Low intensity workouts are better than *nothing at all*; and they may be necessary if you're recovering from injury, or just starting out on the exercise journey.

But once you reach a level of basic fitness, only high intensity (aerobic) workouts will make a difference in terms of your metabolism. High intensity workouts force your body to find energy to help you maintain that level of exercise; and it does so through catabolism.

Myth #4: Too Much Focus

Speeding up your metabolism and achieving your weight loss goals involved a certain degree of focus; after all, there's a lot of things competing for your attention (including that delicious Chef's Special pecan pie!), and you certainly need to be able to keep your eye on the goal in order to maintain your program.

Yet sometimes too much focus can be a bad thing; and some dieters understand this all too well.

Remember: speeding up your metabolism is a *holistic* effort that includes exercise, lifestyle, and diet changes.

Focusing on only one of these at the expense of the others (either one or both) can be detrimental. In fact, in some cases, it can be counter-productive.

So the myth here is that you *shouldn't* go all out and focus on becoming an exercise guru, and then move onto lifestyle, and then to diet.

You have to integrate *all 3* aspects into your life *at the same time*. True, based on your unique situation, you will likely emphasize one more than the others. That's fine and normal. But it's a myth – and a mistake – to ignore any one of these.

It takes all three to speed up your metabolism, and to get you to your weight loss goals for the long-term.

Part 4: Juices That Will Help

DIURETIC JUICES AND BOWEL REGULATORS

Pear Juice With Melon

Ingredients
1 pear
A thick slice of melon
1 bunch of parsley
1 tea spoon of ginger powder (or 1 grated slice)
100 ml of cold water

Preparation
Blend and take immediately.

1 cup

Calories: 70 cal

Coconut Juice

Ingredients
1 cup (200 ml) of coconut water (not the milk but the water inside the coconut) (find it here: www.vitacoco.com)
½ small cucumber

½ carrot
½ apple

Preparation
Blend and take immediately.

1 cup

Calories: 60 cal

Mango Juice With Coconut Water

<u>Ingredients</u>
½ cup plain yogurt skimmed
½ cup of coconut water (not the milk but
the water inside) (find it here:
www.vitacoco.com)
A slice of mango
Cinnamon for sprinkling

Preparation
Blend and take immediately.

1 cup

Calories: 85 cal

Fennel Tea With Orange and Ginger

<u>Ingredients</u>
1 dessert spoon of fennel
Peel of 1 orange

2 cm or 0.8 inch of ginger
1 liter of water

Preparation
Boil the ginger and orange peel for 5
minutes, add the fennel and boil for 3
more. Let it rest for about 10 minutes,
strain and drink.

4 cups

Calories: 0 cal

Watermelon Juice With Celery

Ingredients
1 slice of watermelon
3 stalks of celery, sliced

Preparation
Hit it in the blender and take
immediately.

1 large cup

Calories: 20 cal

_____

Overcoming Abdominal Fat by Carmen Beese